GET HIP!

HOW TO PREPARE FOR AND RECOVER FROM TOTAL HIP REPLACEMENT

ROB TAYLOR &
WAYNE MOSCHETTI, MD, MS

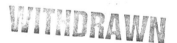

FROG'S LEAP

CONTENTS

INTRODUCTION

How do you know when it's time to get your painful hip replaced?

If you have surgery, how will you feel the next day? After a week? Two weeks? A month?

How soon can you drive a car, cruise through a grocery store? How about ride a bike, play golf, tennis, hike—or ski?

What will the surgery cost?

As an active, 70-year-old facing total hip replacement, I had trouble finding answers to these questions. So I wrote this book.

Mostly it's one man's experience—mine. It's written for people contemplating surgery, not doctors, so I have glossed over some medical complexities. Still, to broaden and deepen my story, I have consulted and cited medical literature, profiled eleven other hip surgery patients, and coaxed insights from my surgeon, who performs hundreds of hip and knee surgeries each year.

This book is about how to prepare for surgery, get home soon, and manage your recovery. It's also a heartfelt tribute to the people who make this surgery possible; they've saved countless people from living on crutches or in wheelchairs.

One cautionary note: my account is not a substitute for professional advice. Any hip-replacement patient should rely primarily on his or her medical team and physical therapist.

Nevertheless, a trip is easier if you have a map—one that shows where you are, where you go next and how you get there. I hope my story will serve as that kind of map. If you're facing hip surgery, it may help you anticipate and understand the path you're traveling—from your first hip pains, through the operating room, to a return to your active life.

To help ease the journey, I've added 18 guidelines; things to keep in mind while following this map.

Hip replacement surgery is commonly hailed as a remarkable success. One study gushed that it is, "widely considered to be one of the most important orthopaedic interventions developed in operative history."[1]

In my case, I had little pain after the surgery. In fact, my hip immediately felt better than it had before the operation. I don't like taking drugs; I took only one mild narcotic pill. I threw out the rest at the local police station. I went home the day after surgery and started physical therapy the next day. I was walking with a cane on the fourth day and taking short hikes in the second week. The walks grew, and after four weeks, my surgeon gave me the green light to do, "anything you feel comfortable doing." I started with golf and moved on to road biking and mountain hiking.

Four months out of the operating room, I figured I was almost back to full strength. My wife and I made plans five months ahead for a 41-mile hike across southern Patagonia's Torres del Paine National Park.

I was lucky. I had advantages to speed my recovery. I started lean and free of health problems; I had anterior surgery, a talented surgeon, a patient physical therapist and a mostly tolerant wife.

My surgeon and physical therapist said my recovery was very good for a person my age. Was it typical? The doctors tell me everyone is different. So I have sprinkled profiles of other hip replacement patients throughout this book. Their stories suggest my recovery wasn't unusual. Of the patients I interviewed, most had experiences like mine. All swore they'd do the surgery again.

"Don't dread the operation," advised one hip arthritis sufferer. "Do what you have to do. You're going to change your life."

To expand beyond anecdotal accounts, I've included references to medical literature. These make up almost all of the 44 footnotes that can be found in the Epilog. These vary from randomized controlled trial studies—the gold standard for medical research—to news stories and product promotions. Though some suggest a medical consensus, no one study should be taken as the final word. As my surgeon put it, paraphrasing Winston Churchill, "doctors rely on medical studies somewhat like a drunk relies on a lamppost, more for support than illumination."

As they say in the drug ads, your results may vary. If you're older, overweight, take narcotic pain medicine before surgery, smoke, or have diabetes or other medical issues, your recovery may take longer than mine. On the other hand, if you're younger, fitter or have better genes, you may leave my rehabilitation in your dust, as did Eric, who is profiled here.

Whatever your condition, I believe the vast majority of hip replacement patients come out ahead. All the patients I have interviewed say they did. Steph got both hips done *twice*, and still suffers from pseudotumors from metal contamination from the first, defective pair of implants. Despite the problems, she declares: "I'm much better off than if I had done nothing."

MY RECOVERY TIMELINE

In short, on the:

- first day after surgery I went home,
- second day, started physical therapy,
- fourth day, walked with a cane, and briefly without one,
- first week, weeded my vegetable garden,
- second week, did short walks,
- third week, drove my car,
- fourth week, walked 1.5 miles and tried chipping and putting,
- fifth week, played 18 holes of golf from a cart,
- eighth week, hiked up a small mountain,
- ninth week, biked ten miles of hills,
- twelfth week, sea-kayaked with orca whales,
- sixteenth week, hiked 7.8 miles up 3,300 ft. to a summit and back.

1

OSTEOARTHRITIS DAWNS

Dogs played leading roles in my hip story. They exposed the ailment—and reaped the benefits of my getting it fixed. I first felt hip pain running on a Virginia forest trail with Gretchen, our chocolate lab, and Maid, our border collie. Chugging down one steep incline, I felt a stab of pain in my right hip. What's that? I asked myself. "That" was arthritis calling.

I was in my mid-60s and had recently retired. I figured the pain would go away. For decades, I had relieved pain in my Achilles tendon by not running for a month or two. So I guessed this hip pain would pass, too.

It didn't. My personal physician, after examining an x-ray, declared I had "osteoarthritis, mild to moderate, on the right side. You've got some in the other hip too," he said, "but not as bad." That wasn't encouraging.

I didn't know it then, but I was running down a path to disability—and an operating room, where, four years later, I would get that right hip replaced.

I was in good company. Almost one in ten adult Americans suffers from osteoarthritis, which some people abbreviate to the initials: OA.[2] In 2010, about 310,800 people in the U.S. 45-years-old or older got total hip replacements. The total hip surgeries had more than doubled in the previous decade, and were forecast to almost double again by 2030.[3,4]

Healthy hip joints are lubricated by a layer of cartilage on the ball-shaped head of the thigh bone (femur). Osteoarthritis arises when the cartilage wears off and/or bone spurs roughen the surface of that ball, causing friction in the socket in which it moves. (For more detail, see: <https://www.arthritis.org/about-arthritis/types/osteoarthritis/what-is-osteoarthritis.php>

Physical Therapy

After my arthritic hip was first diagnosed, a physical therapist gave me some exercises for it—mostly pulling in various ways against big, bright-colored rubber bands. I did the routines for a few months. I cut out running. I turned to biking and golf for exercise. The pain stopped. I had it under control, I thought.

I joined a friend hiking 70 miles of the southern end of the Appalachian Trail. We enjoyed it, and did it again the next year. My wife, Toni, and I enjoyed a three-day "great walk" in New Zealand. For two Julys in a row, I joined neighbors on a 100-mile bike ride to benefit the cancer research institute at the Dartmouth-Hitchcock Medical Center (DHMC) in nearby Lebanon, NH (where I later got my hip replaced). Was I exacerbating my arthritis with exercise? That's not clear. My doctor says light exercise is probably good for OA. But being pain-free was temporary. OA doesn't get better; it usually gets worse. It did for me.

Walking Dogs

In the months following my second year of Appalachian hiking and century biking, the pain started again. Dogs were the immediate cause. I hiked with them daily in the forested hills behind our house in New Hampshire.

By then, Gretchen and Maid had passed on to doggie heaven. But far from relieving my dog walking, that just ramped it up. We got two more border collies, since Toni was into sheepherding. Affectionately known as "Nervous Nelly" and "Hyper Piper", they are the most hyperactive dogs I've ever known.

Piper, rescued from a puppy mill, could never get enough attention or exercise. When I first stepped into her mudroom lair every morning, she leaped into the air for joy and did 360-degree spins until I opened the door to let her outside. Then she and Nelly charged across the front field like race horses breaking out of the starting gate.

Nelly, a three-year-old, had started to mellow, but still had unlimited thirst for hikes. If she saw me lacing up shoes or boots, she moaned and wriggled with anticipation. Piper bounced and spun. If anyone stepped from the house, both dogs sprinted across to the path that led into the forest— only to slink back if we didn't follow. In the woods, they ran like dervishes, but true working dogs, they wouldn't run much past our yard on their own; they waited for Toni or me.

I had stopped jogging because my right hip hurt when I ran. When it started to hurt when I *walked,* I got worried.

With new x-rays, my doctors called it "moderate to severe" arthritis. The x-ray showed the space between the head of my thigh bone (femur) and my socket had shrunk to almost nothing. Most of the cartilage cushion had worn off.

I did a second round of physical therapy. On my physician's suggestion, I used walking sticks for those hour-long dog hikes. In some cases, OA of the hip presents as groin pain. Not mine. It hurt right in the joint itself. But the low level of pain was tolerable. I lived with it.

It's not easy to spot on my x-rays, but the American Academy of Orthopaedic Surgeons has produced the following illustrations to explain the condition:

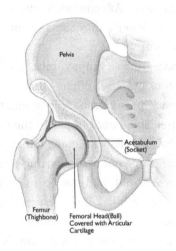

A healthy hip, without osteoarthritis, is cushioned by a smooth lining of cartilage

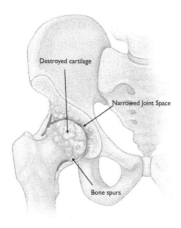

An arthritic hip, showing damage to cartilage and bone
spurs to cause friction in the joint

Images reproduced with permission from OrthoInfo. ©American Academy of Orthopaedic Surgeons. http://orthoinfo.aaos.org.

FOR MORE DETAILED explanation of OA, click on this site offered by the AAOS: https://www.orthoinfo.org/en/diseases--conditions/osteoarthritis-of-the-hip/

Steroid Injections

New Hampshire winter presented a new challenge. I feared the gnawing pain would rear up and bite me on the ski slopes. I love to ski, so I decided to try a steroid injection.

This was not your father's injection. The DHMC performed my "fluoroscopically guided" injection on an x-ray table. The radiologist used x-ray images to get the needle in the right spot: inside the hip capsule. There, the medicine could bathe my arthritic hip joint and hopefully quell some of the pain and inflammation. My doctor said one shot, or a series of them, can provide long-term relief for some people.

Not me. Though initially I skied with only minor pain, the relief wore off in about six weeks—at which point hiking hurt more than before.

Though not impressed with steroids, I went back for more. I had planned a late winter visit with my sister near Aspen. I didn't want to get to Colorado and find that I couldn't ski. Maybe I just needed a second shot to fix my hip, at least temporarily. To make matters worse, my other hip also was giving me a little pain at night. So, when I scheduled a steroid injection again—this time I got shots in *both* hips.

I lucked out. Aspen got blanketed twice with six-to-ten inches of light powder, which is much easier on the legs than hard-packed snow. I skied downhill four days and cross-country one more. Skiing hurt a little, but I was having too much fun to pay heed. I congratulated myself; I could still ski steeps and deeps.

The problem surfaced at the end of each day—when I took off skis and straightened my legs I could barely walk.

GUIDELINE ONE: *Try Alternatives Before the Knife*

My doctors said they wanted me to keep my original hip as long as I could. Physical therapy and steroid injections can delay or even eliminate the need for a hip surgery. They also involve a lot less money and recovery time. Other non-operative options that can help alleviate pain include weight loss and low-impact, light weight-bearing activity like riding a bike or doing water aerobics. But if they don't help, the knife awaits, and is effective.

MEDICAL OPTIONS

By this time, I had plunged hip-deep into the orthopaedic medical world. My first meeting with a hip and knee specialist in New Hampshire had been with a young surgeon at DHMC. Articulate, smart, a graduate of a top medical school, he, I thought, was probably the right guy to operate on my hip—if it came to that.

Though the surgeon had informed me that my arthritis had progressed to "moderate-to-severe," he had stopped short of calling for surgery. That decision was up to the patient, he'd said. He gave me a link to a video that suggested patients try physical therapy and icing, take anti-inflammatory medications and perhaps steroid injections—all before they resorted to the knife. That sounded reasonable.

Now, four months later, I had tried all of the above except surgery. Exercises didn't seem terribly effective. The physical therapist said they would help me to manage or endure the pain; he never suggested that it would go away. The first steroid injection seemed to help for several weeks, but the second pair of shots seemed to have less impact. Neither PT nor steroids had been the solution for me.

From friends, I heard tales of dramatic improvement after hip replacement. Some emerged from surgery saying, "Why didn't I do this earlier?" I watched hip replacement patients dive back into a physical life. One woman I know walked a 10-kilometer race only about four months after replacing *both* hip joints.

Meanwhile, my hip was growing more painful. I relinquished dog hikes to Toni. I was reduced to throwing balls and Frisbees for our high octane canines. I rode my road bike occasionally, but not very far. I wasn't even comfortable playing golf. I hobbled around like Chester on the old television series, "Gunsmoke." And according to Toni, I grew increasingly grouchy.

Okay, I said to myself, I'm ready for surgery. I started reviewing the options.

Total Hip Replacement

The most common repair for arthritic hips is Total Hip Replacement (THR) surgery. THR replaces the ball-and-socket hip joint with artificial implants. Surgeons cut off the head and neck of the thigh bone, or femur. They insert a metal socket into the pelvis, with a plastic, ceramic or metal liner. A matching metal or ceramic ball and metal stem go on the end of the femur.

(For a detailed description of a hip replacement surgery, proceed to Appendix 1.)

Resurfacing

I also considered a wholly different approach: hip resurfacing.

My friend Myles, a veterinary doctor and avid skier, chose to get his femoral heads "resurfaced," instead of replaced. The main advantage, he says, was that surgeons didn't have to cut off the ball-shaped femoral head at the top of his thigh bone. Instead, they reshaped his femoral head ball and cemented on a metal cap, which turned within a metal cup they implanted in his pelvis. If he had a new complication—a femur fracture seemed the nightmare scenario—he'd have more femur left to work with to reconstruct his joint, Myles said.

It sounded promising, but I learned that resurfacing surgeries took longer and put more stress on thigh tissues. Also, some resurfaced joints had caused problems. Resurfacing has tended to use metal-on-metal implants, in which the metal head of the femur turns in a metal cup in the pelvis. The all-metal joints better accommodate the large size of a natural femoral head and offer greater stability and durability, but friction between metal cups and heads sometimes released ions of cobalt and chromium into neighboring tissues and the blood stream. In some patients that triggered multiple afflictions, including fatigue, pain, tissue damage and soft tissue masses called "pseudotumors". These disorders caused metal-on-metal joints and hip resurfacing to fall out of favor. Recently, resurfacing accounted for less than one percent of hip replacement surgeries.[5]

GUIDELINE TWO: *Find a Good, High-volume, Surgeon and Unit*

Studies have demonstrated that hip and knee surgery outcomes tend to be better where surgeons, and hospitals or clinics, do many of these procedures. Some analyses suggest that physicians doing less than 10, and hospitals doing less than 50, total hip replacement operations a year have, on average, higher rates of problems, from dislocations and pulmonary embolisms to deaths.[6,7,8,9,10] Some studies suggest even higher surgical frequency than that would be beneficial. Find out how many hip surgeries are done annually by the surgeon and the medical facilities you are considering. Ask them what percent of their surgery patients have suffered infections (a good goal is less than one percent, my hospital was about 0.3 percent). Also, consult hospital reviews by third parties, but with skepticism; they tend to lack specificity and detail, and may base ratings on easily quantifiable, but irrelevant metrics.

PATIENT #1: MYLES

RESURFACING HIPS

~

Myles is an athletic guy. A one-time college football player, he went on to an active life of tennis and downhill skiing. But in his 60s, arthritic hips slowed him down.

"I was in pain," he recalls, "Walking was difficult. I couldn't bend down and pick up a penny from the ground. Putting on socks or lacing shoes was a challenge."

A doctor of veterinary medicine, Myles had more medical knowledge than most patients. Instead of having total hip replacements, the most common arthritis fix, he chose to have his hips "resurfaced." He liked the idea that this surgery would preserve more of his thigh bones, he said.

Myles did heavy pre-habilitation workouts, mainly aerobic exercises and swimming. He had the hip procedures done in a medical center devoted totally to orthopaedic surgeries. "The fact that there weren't sick people there meant there were less bugs in the hospital," he recalls.

The first hip operation kept him in the medical center one night. He quit pain meds after two days. In about a month, he was walking more than a half-mile; in two months, he was biking; in nine months, he was skiing.

About six years later, he got the second hip done. This time he stayed in the medical center for two nights, largely because of a skin infection for which he was taking antibiotics. But his recovery was equally fast.

One quirk makes his wife smile: occasionally, his hips squeak. "It's always after doing some exercise, when my hip is in a strange position. And it's gone after an hour or two."

Squeaking aside, Myles is pleased with the outcome. He says his metal-on-metal joints have caused no health problems, and to make sure, he gets periodic blood checks for metal leaching. He figures the surgeries achieved 95 percent of his goal to be pain-free and completely mobile. He takes Aleve from time to time for modest pain and inflammation. He's gotten out of the habit of playing tennis, but he's kept skiing—a little more carefully.

∾

FIND A HOSPITAL AND A DOCTOR

Citing illness and liability concerns, I was told, DHMC no longer did hip resurfacing and steered patients to total hip replacement. Myles was skiing well on resurfaced hips, but I went with the local doctors' recommendation. My next challenge was to find the right person and place to do it.

DHMC appeared to be one of the best hospitals in New England, but I hesitated. Should I get this kind of major operation in a regional hospital? I considered going to Boston. The nearest big city, Beantown was bursting with great hospitals, where they surely replaced hips almost as frequently as McDonalds churns out hamburgers.

And what about the surgeon? Myles, my veterinarian buddy, said I should keep down surgical "time, trauma and trash." Translation: get a doctor who works fast, does little tissue damage and avoids infection. Where could I find one who was both well trained and doing a lot of hip surgeries?

The answer to both questions lay close at hand. Three friends of my wife, Toni, had heaped praise on a DHMC surgeon named Wayne Moschetti. I learned that he trained at one of those prestigious Boston hospitals and was performing five hundred knee and hip surgeries each year at a Dartmouth-Hitchcock on a unit dedicated to orthopaedic surgery. (US News & World Report Health rated DHMC as "high performing" in hip replacement, which meant it was in the top 10 percent of hospitals rated. I didn't have much confidence in US News ratings, but it offered some slight comfort.)

Since DHMC and Moschetti met my criteria for surgical training and volume, it seemed to make sense to do the surgery locally; no long drive home, and no long commute for follow-up visits or responding to—heaven forbid—any post-operative problem.

But what about the other surgeon I had met at DHMC? He had seemed impressive. I couldn't find statistics on surgeons' numbers of operations, failure rates and the like. (Local orthopaedic surgeons are listed on several online services, including: <www.orthoinfo.org>, but without data to compare them. Hospitals are rated by several services, but they use metrics that seldom tell you what you want to know.)

I discovered that Moschetti specialized in the direct anterior approach to hip replacement and that the other DHMC surgeon did posterior hip surgeries. My cousin Scott, who had both anterior and posterior hip surgeries, said the anterior technique had led to a faster, less painful recovery. –Advantage Moschetti.

I decided to rely on the old-fashioned interview. I got an appointment to meet Moschetti.

On the appointed day, Moschetti burst into the little examination room for our meeting. Lithe, tall, with an intense look in his dark eyes, he ripped through a quick summary of the surgery. "Any questions?"

Though he seemed in a hurry, I had several. He agreed that the anterior approach generated less pain and sped up the initial recovery, in comparison to the other approaches. He explained how it avoids cutting any muscles. But he added that after about one month there was almost no difference between the outcomes of an anterior or posterior approach. His understated approach appealed to me. I thought anterior surgery, his preferred technique, sounded best; but I liked that he wasn't proselytizing for it.

"I'm ready to schedule surgery." I said. "Will you do it?"

"Meet with my scheduler today," he said. He shook my hand and was gone.

I set a surgery date and left to ski with Myles in Vermont. There was no reason to baby the hip. If I beat it up a little, so what? It was going to be replaced.

CHOOSE A DOOR—FRONT, BACK OR SIDE

For the layman, the choice of total hip replacement (THR) techniques is mostly about how your surgeon cuts into your thigh to get access to the joint. Once they get there, they put in the same kinds of artificial parts. Surgeons tend to get trained on one approach and specialize in it. There are three major approaches:

Posterior Approach—from the back. The most widely used technique, it gives the surgeon broad access to the joint. Surgeons using this back door have to carve through the main butt muscle, the gluteus maximus. This can be done with the grain of the muscle, so it need not be stitched up, but surgeons must cut and separate the muscle to get at the joint where the femur meets the pelvis. They also need to slice the small muscles used to rotate the hip, which they stitch back onto the bone before closing.

Lateral or Anterolateral Approach—from the side. Lateral surgery cuts into the abductor muscle (gluteus medius) to get to the joint, then sews it back together. Lateral hip surgery is associated with a low rate of dislocations after surgery, but due to damage to the muscle—

abductor muscles enable you to move your leg to the side—more lateral patients later suffer from a limp.[11]

Direct Anterior Approach—from the front. The most minimally invasive of the options, it has been associated with the least muscle damage and fast initial recovery. Physicians cut a small window through a thin sheath of fibrous tissue, the fascia, lying over the muscles of the upper thigh. Surgeons insert metal retractors to open a window between muscles —cutting none—to gain access to the joint.[12]

The main advantage of the anterior approach is that it is designed to not cut any muscle, but instead to go between them.[13] Some data would suggest it leads to shorter hospital stays, less pain in the first six weeks and higher activity in the first year after the operation.[14,15] One study showed this technique reduced four-fold the future risk of dislocating the hip, compared to the posterior approach.[16] But medical literature abounds with different findings, and some other studies found little difference for dislocations and only very short-term recovery benefits.

Entering by the front involves some tradeoffs. Though it's easier to get to the hip joint from this side, the opening through which the surgeon operates is smaller, the surgery requires more skill and tends to take a little longer than with posterior entry.[17] There is a risk that the surgeon will hit or stretch a nerve that conveys sensation from the outer thigh, causing numbness or tingling.[18] But posterior entry requires surgeons to detour around the sciatic nerve, so no approach is free of nerve hazards. Some studies have shown anterior surgeries have a slightly higher rate of femur fractures and/or bleeding than the posterior approach. And if anything goes wrong, fixing it is more difficult through the anterior window. But the more experienced the anterior surgeon, the less likely is a complication.

Many anterior hip surgeons use a special table on which the patient's leg is secured to a boom that can be raised, lowered, rotated and pulled as needed. Some surgeons perform anterior hip replacement without such a table, but this usually requires extra help in the operating room to position the leg.

Though the posterior THR remains the most common technique, anterior THR surgery has been gaining a larger share of the hip surgeries since about the year 2000. First described in the 1880's—I dread to think how it turned out back then—it was revived in 1947 by a French surgeon and in the late 1990s by Los Angeles surgeon Dr. Joel Matta.[19]

In his understated fashion, Moschetti was a believer. "The recovery is a little bit quicker, maybe because you're not splitting the g-max (gluteus maximus) and the patient has a little less pain."

"I do 97 percent of my replacements from the anterior approach," he told me.

"Why not all of them?" I asked.

"The posterior is better for certain complicated cases," he said. Those might include patients with large hip deformities, massive bone-loss, surgery requiring significant lengthening of the limb, and overweight patients with a belly fat that could hang over the incision. He figured these didn't include me. I was glad.

Moschetti was careful not to trash-talk the alternatives. His view was that a skilled doctor could be successful using any approach. "The truth of the matter is," he said, "a well done hip replacement through any approach, if you repair the soft tissue structures, things should heal and the patient is going to be happy."

For me, less pain and faster initial recovery made a strong case for the anterior approach. I have to admit, I was also drawn to my surgeon's name—he pronounced it like machete, the two-foot-long blade used to cut sugar cane. I loved the idea that I could say I fixed my hip with a Moschetti.

(Moschetti confessed that "machete" was the Americanized pronunciation. The correct Italian pronunciation was "MO-SKETTI", which takes the drama out of it.)

A nurse was unimpressed that I liked the surgeon's name; she said I could have been sent to Dr. Slaughter.

You Have to Wait

I was ready to climb up on the operating table, but it wasn't ready for me. Moschetti's backlog of cases was about six weeks, so I was looking at May Day as my target for the new hip. That might mean golf in June, I figured.

The scheduler had other ideas. Steroids tend to suppress the immune system. She said they don't do surgeries less than three months after the last injection. Moschetti told me that some data would suggest you should wait up to a year after a steroid injection before surgery. After I gave her the date of my last steroid shot, she put me down for the hip replacement May 24. I'd have to put up with my bum hip for three extra weeks. Golf would have to wait for July.

*GUIDELINE THREE: **Check the Approach***

Some studies have found anterior hip surgeries tend to give the patient less pain and a quicker initial recovery than the other alternative approaches (anterolateral, lateral, and posterior). My cousin, who had an anterior approach on one side and a posterior approach on the other, agreed. So did my surgeon and my physical therapist. Also, patients opened by the other approaches may endure short-term bans on certain movements, such as crossing their legs or bending the joint more than 90 degrees.

PATIENT #2: SCOTT

"GO ANTERIOR"

~

My cousin Scott's hips went bad in his 50s. "I was taking 800 mg. of ibuprofen a day," he recalls, "I was limping and walking bent over. It was totally bone-on-bone on my left side... People were saying, 'you ought to do something about it.'"

"I finally said, 'enough is enough.'"

First, Scott tried injections of rooster comb tissues (currently not recommended by the American Academy of Orthopaedic Surgeons). The x-ray-guided procedure aimed to put some padding between the ball and socket of his left hip. It was supposed to last six to eight weeks. Scott's pain was back in ten days.

His doctor proposed resurfacing his hip. But once the surgeon opened the joint from the posterior approach, he found nodules on Scott's femur he didn't like. Instead of reshaping and capping the femoral head, he did a total hip replacement.

Scott got the second hip done a year later by anterior

entry. This time he was able to sleep on his side the first night home, rather than waiting ten days for pain to ease, as after the posterior hip replacement.

Regardless of surgical technique, Scott wasted no time getting back to his life. Using a wooden walking stick, he started going back to his office a week after the first hip surgery, and four days after the second. He ignored doctors' warnings to wait six weeks to drive; he drove after five days. He hit the treadmill at the gym after three weeks, and moved on to elliptical striders.

Years later, Scott is doing everything he used to do before his hips went bad: skiing, playing tennis, golf and paddleball. He's more agile and flexible moving around big sailboats.

He expects his artificial hip joints will wear out before he does. But he believes the surgery will keep getting faster and better. "The next time I go in, it will probably be an outpatient surgery. And it will last me the rest of my life."

Scott is a fan of anterior hip surgery. Compared to his posterior surgery, he had less pain, his scar was smaller, his recovery faster and his range of motion greater. "If I have to do it again, they're going to do it in the front," he says.

∾

5

SURGERY PREPARATION

Aperennial optimist, I had already put down a deposit on a five-day, August sea-kayaking trip at Johnstone Strait, where killer whales frolic in the northern gateway to Vancouver, B.C. and Puget Sound. By August, I had figured, I should be ready for anything. But as I read more, I grew alarmed by stories of people who were painfully disabled for months. I started worrying that I might not recover enough by August to paddle a kayak. The trip would come 12 weeks after surgery, the week before a Seattle-area wedding that Toni, my son Grant, and I planned to attend.

In my last pre-operative meeting, I demonstrated for Moschetti the seated position I'd use to paddle a kayak. "Will I be able to do it?" I asked.

"You should be fine," he reassured me. "You may need to take some ibuprofen."

I didn't want to leave anything to chance. Everything I heard and read suggested that I should work on fitness *before* the operation. The fitter you go in, some said, the faster you will recover.

Prehablitation

My hospital gave me a loose-leaf binder of documents that included one page of exercises to be performed by hip and knee patients while in the hospital, recovering from surgery. The majority was designed to be performed in bed; the most aggressive being the "inner-thigh squeeze," which called for compressing a pillow between your knees. A few called for sitting in a chair and alternatively straightening your leg and pulling it back. These were not going to get me fit before I went under the knife.

I found a little more on the Internet. Alberta, Canada, posted a set of pre-operative exercises, as did one health blog. Both were designed to prepare a patient for hip replacement surgery, but both suffered some of the same shortcomings as my binder's exercises—they were mostly done in a prone or sitting position. They were, to be blunt, a little wimpy.

So I developed my own pre-habilitation workouts. Some I based on the physical training I had done when I first reported my hip pain. Many of these called for pulling against elastic bands. I also found exercise machines at my gym that resisted opening my thighs and squeezing them together. I used a leg-press, stationary bicycle, and various machines for upper body strength.

My son, Grant, talked me into swimming. I got hooked and worked up to swimming laps about a half-hour at a time, alternating strokes. I swam like a brick, but kicking water seemed a great low-impact hip exercise. It also gave me a full body workout and better aerobic exercise than anything else I tried.

Surgery 101 Class

A couple of weeks before my surgery date, Dartmouth-Hitchcock called me in for an hour-long briefing for knee and hip surgery candidates. A half-dozen of us sat around a conference table. Nicole explained the techniques of knee and hip surgeries and what we needed to know to prepare for them.

Much attention focused on precautions against infection, which was said to occur in only 1-to-3 percent of hip surgeries, generally, but was about one in 300 at DHMC. The hospital proposed to give us antibiotic nasal cream to rub in our nostrils for several days before surgery to eradicate MRSA, an antibiotic-resistant staphylococcus bacteria. We would also get anti-bacterial soap to scrub with the night before and day of surgery. The night before surgery, we should sleep in freshly washed sheets and bedclothes and keep dogs out of the bedroom.

My procedure, including anesthesia, was supposed to take about an hour and a half. Afterward, I'd get moved to a hospital room. I'd wear inflatable leg-compression devices on my calves during surgery and for hours after, to keep blood moving out of my lower legs and help prevent blood clots. I'd be on antibiotics for 24 hours and blood thinners for 30 days. The typical patient spends between one and two days in the hospital, they said. After release, they warned patients not to drive a car until they were off narcotics and four-to-six weeks out of surgery.

I had heard that with lower levels of anesthesia, some people got released from the hospital the day of surgery. That sounded great to me; cut Medicare's bill, get away from antibiotic-resistant bacteria at the hospital and start rehab that much sooner. I asked for minimal anesthesia and a same-day release. The answer: maybe. At the time, Medicare did not consider hip replacement an outpatient surgery. But if, after admission to the hospital, you meet all of the discharge criteria for a safe release, sometimes the hospital will send you home.

Forms, Forms, Forms

The surgery briefing was only the first of four appointments the hospital scheduled for me that day, back-to-back. In the second, a doctor grilled me about my medical history; his job was to uncover any problems that might complicate surgery, such as allergies, heart problems or diabetes, which I fortunately didn't suffer. In the third, the "orthopaedic care manager" discussed surgery timing and details and fielded questions. This was probably where people taller than six feet might request an extra-long hospital bed. I didn't need it. The final session took me to a lab to give a blood sample for analysis.

At the hospital's request, I sent in a copy of my advance directive. It expressed my wishes that doctors not make extreme measures to keep me alive if I became incurably sick and unable to speak for myself. It also gave Toni my authorization to make decisions for me about such things, as well as legal power to act in my stead, if I became incapacitated. Of course, none of us expected any of these situations to develop during my hospitalization for hip replacement. But there's always a risk—albeit small—of something going drastically wrong during major surgery. So it seemed a good idea for the hospital to have that document on file.

Not all forms were so useful. I got a series of forms to fill out for each appointment. Each time I was asked to fill out the same multi-page Medicare form, which asked if I had black lung disease, end stage renal disease, was a veteran, was treating a work-related injury, an accidental injury, and the like. It even asked the exact dates I and my wife retired. I didn't mind filling it out once, or even once a day. But on the four-appointment day I was required to fill out the same form four times. I explained to a receptionist that my information had not changed in the last hour.

Protests were useless. I was told, "Medicare requires it."

GUIDELINE FOUR: Exercise Before Surgery

If your doctor doesn't recommend a workout regimen, find one online. Studies show that people who do physical therapy before surgery recover faster.

Guideline Five: Find out What Will Happen in the Hospital and After

You should get an extensive briefing or detailed information on what to expect at the hospital, how to get yourself in shape for surgery, and how to prepare your home for your initial recovery, which is in the next chapter.

6

PREPARING FOR IMMOBILITY

The instructions for patients returning from surgery called for a bedroom to be accessible without stairs. Fortunately, our bedroom is on the first floor. But that was just the first of several issues on my to-do list. My loose-leaf binder on surgery said I needed an array of gear to prepare for the operation.

The nearby Bugbee Senior Center said it would loan me most of the big stuff: a cane, crutches, a shower seat and a walker. What a nice service! They merely asked that I return them when I was done.

I realized that I might need several other gadgets:

- a dressing stick, with hooks that you use to pull on pants when you can't reach past your knee;
- a plastic sock puller, to pull a sock over your feet with cords (same reason);
- a three-foot-long "grabber" to pick up things from the ground;
- a long-handled shoehorn;

- and a leg-lifting strap, to hoist your bad leg onto
  a bed or couch after surgery.

I got almost all from an online vendor in a combination hip surgery kit that also included a sponge on a long handle. I added a travel vest with many pockets, which I happened to have. When I was hobbling on crutches or a walker, the vest could carry all kinds of things, from glasses to books. My binder called for a raised toilet seat, but our hospital surgery briefer had said we didn't really need that.

The Race to Prepare

I figured I would be immobile for at least a week after surgery, and unable to drive for weeks, so as the date approached, I tried to get chores done and supplies stocked so I wouldn't leave Toni any more tasks than necessary. It was spring in New England. Toni lined up people to mow grass and help in the garden while I couldn't. Meanwhile, I:

- mowed and weed-whacked around the house,
- bought extra food—40-to-50 lb. bags—for border
  collies and chickens,
- stocked up a two-month supply of toilet paper
  and paper towels,
- picked up three or four frozen dinners,
- planted the last of my vegetable garden,
- cleaned out our fireplace and moved indoor
  firewood supplies outdoors,
- replaced flannel sheets with linen sheets on
  guest beds,
- got a haircut, and,
- put another "super" box of empty honeycomb on
  top of my bee hive, in hopes that my bees would
  fill it.

Practice Being an Invalid

I rehearsed lifting my right leg with a strap as I got out of bed, sleeping on my back and walking on crutches. What about going to the bathroom to pee? As an older man with an enlarged prostate, I had been making that trek about three times a night. The doctor who checked my fitness for surgery suggested, "Use a urine jug." So, I practiced that, too, with interesting results.

I placed an empty plastic juice bottle next to my bedside table. Waking up that night, I rolled over on my side and felt around until I found the jug. I screwed off the top and tried to slip my penis in. The opening was larger than a pop bottle's top, but not large enough. I couldn't get the head of my unit inside without plugging the mouth and risking a urine explosion. Still, in the dark room I somehow managed to hold the tip of my little organ on the lip of the bottle and pee flowed in. I screwed on the top, congratulated myself, and went back to sleep.

The second pee didn't go so well. I tried to tip the bottle, now holding more than a cup of fluid, so I could pee into it again without spilling or climbing out of bed. I maneuvered close to the edge of the bed, leaning on my arthritic hip, so the bottle could hang off on an angle. But I didn't get close enough. As I tried perching my penis on the open top, working by feel in the dark, some urine poured out onto the bed.

End of experiment.

I got up, screwed the top back on the bottle, and walked to the bathroom.

In the morning, I found plenty of pee in the bottle, easing my embarrassment somewhat. I found another bottle that seemed had a bigger mouth. The label read, "Only Lemonade." I etched "NOT" in black above the label (to prevent it being mistaken for lemonade). But when I tried it the second night, I dropped the screw cap, which clattered across the floor in the dark. The hell with the bottle, I said to myself, and walked to the bathroom.

When I told Toni about my jug adventures, she rolled her eyes and muttered that I was getting a little "obsessive."

Long after, I discovered that various urine jugs are sold on the Internet, with large mouths for men, "ladies' adaptors" for women and interestingly, one product claimed a "spill-proof cap." I wondered how that might work.

As my surgery approached, my hip pain got worse. It woke me up several times a night. I often rose before 6 a.m. because the hip was keeping me awake. Bottle or not, I was ready to slice up that hip.

GUIDELINE SIX: *Gather Gear You'll Need*

You will need some things to help you get through the first few weeks of playing semi-invalid. Some of the gear may be available for lending from a senior center. Others may be available to be ordered as a package.

7

GAME ON—MY SURGERY

I am checking in at the reception desk. Moschetti appears next to me in blue scrubs. He's smiling broadly.

"We're ahead of schedule," he says. "I've done two cases and we're ready for you. Let me lead you back."

Hastily, I sign a few forms and hobble down the hall after the tall figure in blue scrubs. A nurse takes over getting me in the hospital gown. I struggle to tie the strings behind my head.

"Ready?" An intern or resident introduces himself. Another young, athletic-looking guy. A middle-aged man comes in. "I'm Brian Sites. I'm going to be your anesthesiologist. Shall we discuss your options?"

"I think we've already settled on a spinal block and sedation," I say. I am sure I don't want general anesthesia, which I think would mean a longer recovery. "And I request that you go light with the sedation."

"Okay," he says. He proceeds to explain how the spinal block and the sedation work, and the long list of things that could go wrong, the kind of spiel that US doctors and drug ads on TV say to keep their malpractice lawyers happy. You could wind up permanently damaged or dead, but such outcomes are rare.

The spinal injection should temporarily eliminate feeling from both my legs, he explains, but I would be breathing on my own. Sedation should make me sleepy, which could be deep or shallow, but not out cold. Complete unconsciousness with a breathing tube in place and a machine breathing for me would be general anesthesia. I repeat that I don't want that.

Another guy in scrubs enters and introduces himself as the assistant anesthesiologist. The little dressing room is getting crowded. I am asked my name and date of birth. Someone asks which hip is getting replaced, and marks that side with green ink.

I can't resist telling the story about the guy who got the wrong leg amputated, only to be returned to surgery to take off the other leg that should have been amputated the first time. The patient sued, I explain, but the judge threw out his case, saying he didn't have a leg to stand on.

They must not have heard that one, because I got some worried looks followed by nervous chuckles. Surgical mistakes are no joke.

"Ready to go?" I lie down on the table in the dressing room. They give me a pill and wheel me out. My mind is already getting a little foggy. At some point, they sit me up and stick a needle in my back for the spinal anesthesia, to block pain from my legs. Aside from that, Sites gives me only Versed, an anti-anxiety medication, like Valium, that makes me drowsy and light-headed, but not unconscious. The sedative tends to impair recall, so from there, my recollection is spotty, but here's what I do remmber:

On the Table

Special padded boots are placed on my feet (they look like ski boots) and I am transferred to a special operating table. The next thing I recall is the whirring of a drill, with pressure on my pelvis. I ponder. That must be Moschetti reaming out the worn-out cartilage in my pelvis, the acetabulum. I don't recall his sawing off the end of my femur and the dislocation of the femur ball from the joint. Or maybe I just lost the memory. That's just as well. I remember hearing the tap, tap, tap, which I figure is Moschetti hammering the implant into my open femur. Or was it the cup? Or did I dream all of it? I don't know.

My memories fade in and out. Someone sews up inside the wound and closes the outer layer of skin with glue and tape. I'm done. Nurses wheel me to a "post-anesthesia" recovery area, where I fall asleep.

Toni has settled into the waiting room. An electronic board shows the number assigned to me—like an arriving airline flight listed on an airport monitor. When the light next to my number flashes on "recovery", she knows I am out of surgery.

In the Post Anesthesia Care Unit, Moschetti tells her it has been a "textbook" operation. One of the anesthesiologists says I had talked to the surgeons throughout the procedure.

Titanium, Ceramic and Plastic

Later, Moschetti told me my skinny hip made his job easy; he completed the operation in 69 minutes, compared to his average 78. In my pelvis, he put a metal cup with no screw holes and a plastic liner, matched up with a ceramic head on a titanium stem, mounted in my femur. The surface of both the cup and stem have a porous metal coating that invites bone to grow into the pores. They will become a part of my skeleton.

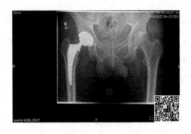

My new parts

Guideline Seven: What kind of anesthesia?

A study of more than 20,000 cases that found patients with spinal anesthesia spent less time in the operating room, recovery room and the hospital, compared to patients with general anesthesia. But medical studies give conflicting conclusions. It's up to the patient and doctors to pick what's best. I was surprised to learn that recovery from general anesthesia may be faster than from spinal anesthesia and sedation. But the 20,000-case study and others convinced me that the spinal is marginally safer. Which makes sense, since a general takes you to the verge of death and holds you there until they bring you back. That study found a spinal nerve block is associated with lower rates of adverse events, including heart attacks, strokes, and ventilator use.[20]

8

GETTING ON MY FEET

W hen I came to, Toni sat next to the bed, looking concerned. I was in a hospital room. Nurses cycled through, introducing themselves. One couldn't find a body temperature. She tried at least three thermometers. Finally, she concluded I was about three degrees Celsius too cold. Nurses piled heated blankets all over me and around my head. I felt like an Egyptian mummy. Was it time to put me in a sarcophagus?

Toni looked stricken. My color had turned gray, she said later, but it didn't last. In an hour, my temperature rose. I felt warmer. Gray seeped out of my face. Toni started to relax.

I slept much of the day, interrupted by nurses with drugs or food or blood-pressure cuffs and thermometers.

I wasn't in much pain, which surprised me. They had carved up my hip and reassembled it with metal and plastic, and the pain was less than I had felt for the last month. Was that due to pain meds or Moschetti's injecting local anesthetic in the wound? I didn't know.

Late in the day, I tried to stand. I sat on the side of the bed facing a walker. I put weight on my stocking feet and slowly stood up. I wanted to walk a little, but I felt dizzy. I was afraid I might faint if I tried walking. With the nurse's encouragement, I settled back onto the bed.

Shaky Start

I had hoped to be released from the hospital the day of the surgery. I had given up that dream because Toni had a theater rehearsal that evening. It now appeared that I wouldn't have gotten out anyway. To get released, I needed to show I could pee, walk around with a walker or crutches, climb up and down stairs and maintain stable vital signs, like temperature, heart rate and blood pressure. My temperature and heart rate were okay, but otherwise I was checking "none of the above."

The next day—my second in hospital—did not start well. I had slept pretty well, but the first blood pressure test registered only in the mid-90s for the systolic (higher) number; which was too low. And instead of rising towards my normal 120, my systolic pressure fell, first to 84, then 86. Nurses frowned. I also couldn't pee. "The bladder is usually the last to wake up," a nurse said. Nurses drained my bladder by pushing a catheter into my penis, which was not fun. Did I mention that one sheds all dignity when one dons a hospital gown?

Cousin Scott recommends requesting catheterization while under sedation, before surgery, and leaving it there until the next day. Pulling it out then "is less painful and quicker" than putting it in and withdrawing it the second day, he says.

Oh no, I thought: not only did I fail to get out the day of surgery, I'm not going to get out the next day. But my condition turned around. In retrospect, I figure I was dehydrated. I drank lots of water. A little after noon, my blood pressure climbed to 97 over 40-something. One nurse suggested that was good enough for me to leave.

Still, my urinary tract had yet to wake up. I managed to pee about 275 ccs, without a catheter. (I muttered "eureka" over my urethra). But an ultrasound probe showed I had 400 ccs more in my bladder. Probably not enough "voiding" to be confident they could send me home, one nurse said. (If I couldn't pee at home, urine buildup could overstretch my bladder, and they'd drag me back to the hospital.)

A physical therapist led me through the post-operative exercises that people can do in the hospital: squeeze buttocks, flex quadriceps, squeeze a pillow between your knees, slide your heel forward and back; and from a seated position, lift your leg horizontal and pull it back toward your butt. Some of these hurt my carved-up leg. I did not complain that they were wimpy.

The therapist was about to take me on a walker stroll around the ward when I blurted, "I think I need to pee," took the jug and shuffled into the bathroom.

I stood there, holding the jug over the toilet. Minutes passed. I felt a slight burning sensation in my urethra. I looked down and saw the most beautiful yellow liquid. I emerged with a trophy jug of about 500 ccs.

"I think you're going to get released today," said one of the nurses.

Released

They let me go. The breakthrough came about 24 hours after I came out of surgery. Aside from urinating, I demonstrated that I could shuffle on crutches around the ward and up and down stairs. My blood pressure reached a normal range.

I had been sharing the room with a man who had got a titanium bar inserted in his femur. He was shuffling around the ward on a walker, but hadn't been able to pee much yet. Nurses made him stay another night. He was disappointed.

I didn't realize until later how fortunate I was. Dartmouth Hitchcock had been releasing most of their hip replacement patients after one or two nights in the hospital. But a major study found that in 2010 the average length of stay nationally was "just under four days."[21] Several studies showed the lengths of stay were shrinking. One national study found the mean hospital stay shrank to a little under three days in 2013.[22]

My tolerant Toni picked up my medications from the hospital and the last of my gadgets from the Bugbee Center. A nurse pushed me in a wheelchair down to the North Entrance, where Toni was waiting with her Subaru. I hobbled out on my crutches—free at last.

GUIDELINE EIGHT: *Get Out of the Hospital Soon*

A quick release from the medical center has many advantages. General hospitals tend to host bacteria, including drug-resistant strains, that you want to avoid. Studies show that the faster a patient gets physically active, the better the outcome. Longer hospital stays have been linked to greater risk of complications and hospital readmissions. And of course, additional days in a hospital drive up the cost to patient and insurer. One study put the cost of one extra day at $2,900.[23,24] Medicare and hospitals are trying to cut the length of stay of hip replacement patients. Some even get released on the day of surgery.

Guideline Nine: Prepare the Car

Climbing into a vehicle can be awkward after surgery, especially posterior surgery. It's usually helpful to slide the front passenger seat all the way back and recline the backrest a little. If you're the patient, get to where your back is facing the seat, then lower your butt onto it, using crutches or a walker and the doorway for support. Push back with your good leg, then lift both legs into the car, turning them toward the front. If the car is low-slung and you find this difficult, you may want to put a pillow on the seat to raise it.

PATIENT #3: SANDI

THR AS OUTPATIENT SURGERY

~

S andi is a model patient. When she got her hip replaced in her mid-50s, she went home from the hospital the same day. Seven months later she was waterskiing.

Sandi's recovery was smooth. She used only three of her Tramadol narcotic pain pills. She walked with a cane in less than a week and was walking a half-mile within two or three weeks.

She looked back nine months later with satisfaction. "I don't have pain in my hip. It doesn't hold me back from anything."

She credited her recovery to faithful performance of exercises her physical therapist assigned. "I did what they told me to do. They said, 'don't do more.' So, I kind of held back." After about one month she started working out, carefully, on an elliptical exerciser in her home.

No stranger to exercise, Sandi had played softball for years and grew up to be an avid skier, until pain in her left hip forced her to give that up. Before surgery, walking around her neighborhood became a chore. She couldn't even walk up stairs or sleep through the night without pain.

She tried yoga, physical therapy and acupuncture; none proved effective. Her daughter, who worked as an orthopaedic nurse at DHMC, talked her into seeing Dr. Moschetti. He saw no point in trying steroid injections, and scheduled her for a hip replacement, she said. "It was inevitable that it was going to have to be replaced."

While her recovery went well, it was not unusual—except for the same-day release from the hospital. For that, her daughter proved to be her ace in the hole. Sandi was scheduled first in line for that day's surgery, and by 6 p.m. she demonstrated she could shuffle around with a walker. Her daughter took her home and supervised her medications.

~

9

FIRST NIGHT HOME

As Toni drove me away from the hospital, my hip felt pretty good. It was just a little sore under the waterproof bandage covering my incision.

Earlier, I had watched a woman on YouTube say that after anterior hip replacement she hadn't even needed anything stronger than Tylenol for pain. I had doubted it at the time; but now it sounded possible.

Arriving home, I used crutches to climb out of the car and up the mudroom steps. I opened the door. Nelly and Piper ran past, then turned back to investigate why I had grown two additional metal legs. Nelly cowered. Piper leaped up and down. (fortunately, not on me; it would not be good to get knocked over on my new hip.)

Toni parked, brought in my hospital overnight bag, a sack full of medicines and the walker. Our wonderful neighbor Carolyn Mertz had dropped off a delicious dinner of chicken and kale salad. I ate with gusto, took my evening meds and hobbled into our bedroom. I gingerly stripped off clothing and climbed into bed. We'd done it!

Can I Sleep?

I had read that after the operation I'd have to sleep on my back, be very careful not to cross my legs or bend my surgical leg more than 90 degrees from my upper body, and always put a pillow between my knees if I rolled on my side. It sounded like my night would be ruled by Nurse Ratched from "One Flew Over the Cuckoo's Nest."

In fact, *none* of that applied to me. Those precautions were for posterior surgery patients, said the therapist at the hospital. Anterior approach patients can sleep any way they like, she said. Which was good to hear, as I was a restless sleeper. That night, I vacillated between lying on my back and on my left side, on the uncut hip.

I took one of the Tramadol pills from the hospital and slept. When I awoke a little after midnight to a full bladder I didn't bother with the "NOT Only Lemonade" bottle. I pushed the walker into the bathroom and leaned on it until I was finished peeing. I did the same thing about 4 a.m. The next day I discarded the pee bottle, to Toni's relief.

Drugs

As I expected, the hospital recommended a long list of drugs:

- Tramadol, 50 mg., was the only opioid pain reliever, and came with the instructions, take "as needed." Instructions for this drug included the warning, "**MISUSE OF NARCOTIC PAIN MEDICATION CAN CAUSE ADDICTION, OVERDOSE, OR DEATH.**" I was into minimizing, so I figured I would not take it unless the pain mounted high or kept me awake.

-Aspirin, 81mg. (formerly called baby aspirin). I was supposed to take it twice a day as a blood thinner, to prevent clotting. One of the more serious complications of hip surgery was the risk of a clot forming in the leg and finding its way to a lung (pulmonary embolism), which could be fatal.

-Naproxen, aka Aleve, 500 mg., anti-inflammatory, the generic version of Aleve. I was to take one tablet twice a day with meals "for 41 days."

-Omeprezole, aka Prilosec, 20 mg. It was recommended once a day in the morning to protect the stomach lining from other meds that would assault it.

-Senna-ducosate 8.6, aka Pericolace, 50 mg. Two tablets twice a day would "maintain normal bowel pattern while taking narcotic pain medication."

-Acetaminophen, aka Tylenol, 500 mg. I was supposed to take two tablets every 8 hours for about a week, then as needed for pain. My personal physician said this would put less strain on my liver than the anti-inflammatories and opioid.

-Polyethylene glycol, aka Miralax, 17 g. was added for me to use if I had trouble with constipation.

I had drug benefits with Humana, which meant going to Wallmart's pharmacy to fill prescriptions. But Dartmouth-Hitchcock was able to order them from Wallmart for me. Toni had picked up a bulging bag of pill bottles at the hospital for me as I was checking out.

Getting Comfortable

My first full day home I awoke feeling grateful. I had a little pain and swelling under my incision, but it was less than I had felt daily before surgery.

Most of the patients I interviewed reported similarly low levels of pain—2-3 on a 10-point scale—for the first week after surgery. One friend got teary when he awoke after his operation; it was the first time in months that he felt no acute hip pain.

Though I used the walker to get to the bathroom at

night, I found forearm-crutches more convenient for hobbling around the house. I soon discovered that I could carry things in my right hand and rely only on the left crutch to help shift weight off my right leg.

I gulped down my medications and breakfast and took up residence with my computer on a comfortable chair. Let the recovery begin.

10

FIRST PHYSICAL THERAPY

Easy Does It

About 10 a.m. my second morning home Toni dropped me off for my first session at BE Fit Physical Therapy. I was eager to start aggressive rehabilitation exercises. David Barlow, my therapist, had other ideas.

"You've gotta give it time to heal," he said. "If you push it you'll just make the healing process take longer."

David reviewed the exercises the hospital recommended —all pretty wimpy. He urged me to go easy on them for a few days or even the first week. Not too long ago, hip replacement patients didn't even come in to see him until six weeks after surgery, he said. The schedule had moved up with anterior surgeries, but he suggested I was starting too soon. We agreed I'd come back the next week.

I returned to my easy chair. When the leg felt swollen and sore, I lay down on a sofa with my feet up on a pillow. An ice bag helped reduce the swelling. I napped an hour or two on the sofa for the first few days. I rose to do a lap around the house on crutches. I even found I could throw a ball for the dogs outside, leaning on one crutch and using a long-handled ball chucker. I did light PT exercises about three times a day, but not aggressively.

Toni made me dinner at home my second night home. The next, we drove to a friend's house for dinner. I was happy to call it a night about 9 p.m., go home and slip into bed. Though the therapist had said I didn't need the leg-lifting strap, I found it useful for climbing into bed. Hoisting the leg without it sometimes hurt.

GUIDELINE TEN: *Do Your PT*

Hospitals are starting to send patients home with a written guide to exercises they can and should do, without supervision, to restore their hip and leg muscles. But a physical therapist can show you how to strengthen muscles and expand the range of motion of your joint, while making adjustments for the varying responses and exercise skills of individual patients. He or she is also a useful sounding board as to what pain is normal and what you should be able to do and when.

DISCOMFORT

Constipation
On my third night home, my stomach blew up like a balloon. Abdominal pain woke me in the middle of the night. I wondered if I'd need to go back to the hospital.

I thought it was just constipation. I had got Toni to pick up a backup anti-constipation drug, Miralax. I'd taken it the previous afternoon, but my discomfort was sharp and growing.

Hobbling out to my drug stockpile, I reviewed my instructions. Sure enough, I had under-dosed myself with the original stool softener. I had been taking one tablet twice a day, instead of the recommended two. Could that be why I was having trouble? On the other hand, my instructions said that the stool softener was to reduce constipation from the opioid drug, of which I had only taken one tablet. So why was I feeling like I might explode?

Whatever the cause, I needed to do something about it. Early the next morning I took two of the softeners and another dose of the Miralax, along with my other drugs.

Relief came a few hours later. The moral of that story is, read your drug instructions carefully.

Swelling, etc.

My right thigh was swelling a bit. I treated that by lying down and elevating my legs on a pillow. A couple of times a day I put an ice bag on the leg and moved it around for an hour or so. That seemed to make the leg feel better and the swelling recede.

The hospital had warned against deep vein thrombosis, a blood clot that can lead to a pulmonary embolism. Even before I left the hospital, I felt a pain in my left chest, which went away soon. A sharp pain recurred in the same area about 24 hours after I got out of the hospital, then disappeared again. At least one more time I felt pain in the same general area. It occurred to me that it could be an embolism, but since it kept going away, I rejected the idea. It was one of those pains that one never knows how to explain. Later, I read that pulmonary embolism, while serious, is extremely rare. One large study found it happened in less than half of one percent of hip replacement patients.[25]

*GUIDELINE ELEVEN: **Read Drug Instructions Carefully***

It's easy to overdose or under-dose medications. Read the instructions more than once to make sure you don't miss anything —as I did.

PATIENT #4: NEIL

BACK TO THE MOUNTAINS

~

Retired in his late 60s, Neil was out climbing mountains most weekends in the Cascade Range of Washington and Oregon—until arthritis in his right hip slowed him down.

As a hiking fanatic, Neil was known for the loads he carried and the crooks in his legs. I once climbed Mt. Rainier with him, and fondly remember seeing the peak framed by his bowed legs as he strode up the mountain ahead.

Alas, hiking became painful, and in 2012, Neil interrupted the hikes to replace his right hip.

After lateral surgery, his doctors had him stay three nights in the hospital. Though that was longer than most patients I interviewed, his recovery accelerated. He was comfortable walking with a cane in about five days and was taking walks without a cane in a week.

Neil's measure of the surgery was how quickly he got back on the trails.

"I waited about five weeks before taking my first modest hike, one of about six miles with 2,000 feet of elevation gain," says Neil. (Some people would call that a serious hike.) "After that I was back to regular hiking, although I didn't take my first multi-day backpacking trip until five months after the surgery."

Neil's doctor told him to cut out running, and he reluctantly complied. The physician also told him to keep his backpack weight under 50 pounds, "which I've probably exceeded a few times," Neil allows.

His hiking legs are not perfect. When descending steep slopes under a backpack, he says, he feels the impact in his new right hip, though "nothing that I would call pain." His left knee has become increasingly weak and aches after a hike. One doctor theorizes that by unconsciously favoring the right hip, to protect it, he has placed extra strain on the left knee. Pain is starting to crop up in the other knee too, particularly after descending steep slopes. So, Neil is turning his attention to the knees. Last I heard, he was considering trying a steroid injection before weighing knee surgery.

∼

12

ADJUSTING TO THE NEW HIP

Sleeping
  My hospital's therapist said that after an anterior hip replacement I didn't need a pillow between my legs if I slept on my side. But I felt more secure using a pillow. So I settled into a pattern. I placed a bed pillow next to the bed. I tried to sleep on my back, usually without success. Eventually I picked up a pillow, jammed it between my legs and turned to sleep on the side of my "good" hip.

I found it easier to sleep on my side. I soon progressed to using a thin seat cushion between my knees, instead of the pillow. And since pain stabbed my hip when I started climbing into bed, for the first week I used the leg-lifter for that.

I have long been a restless sleeper. I shift position several times a night. That didn't change. In the first weeks after surgery, I usually awoke at least three or more times a night. Sometimes I got out of bed, shuffled my walker to the bathroom and peed. Sometimes I just changed my position, going from my side to my back and, after a few minutes, reverting to my side. In a few weeks, I could also sleep on my stomach.

Cramps

Nobody warned me about cramping. When I shifted from my side to my back, straightened legs and slid my feet down, the quadriceps muscles down the front of my thighs cramped spasmodically. I learned to reduce the cramping by straightening the leg very slowly, but I couldn't eliminate it.

The first time this happened, I stifled a yelp of pain and surprise. The cramps were hard to control, fairly painful, and my hamstrings often joined in the fun. Muscles on the front and back of my thigh fought for supremacy. I was unsure how to combat them. With my hip soreness, I had to be careful about how I responded to the cramps, for fear of hurting the new joint. As I grew accustomed to this, I suppressed the yelp, managed the cramps and lived with them. Moschetti told me that dehydration could produce cramping, so I tried to drink more. In time, the cramps faded away.

I Can Walk!

I first caught myself walking on my fourth day out of the hospital. I was beginning to use a cane or one crutch in my left hand to give stability to my steps in the house. I was shuffling around the kitchen, moving plates onto the table and back to the counter, using one crutch. At some point, I realized that I had just schlepped a plate to the counter without using the crutch.

Toni sat at our breakfast table, reading the news online.

"Look at this," I said, as I walked slowly past the table.

"At what?" she asked.

"No crutches," I said.

"Oh, you're walking!" she said. "But honey, please don't do that. You don't want to push the leg while it's healing."

I agreed. I picked up my crutch.

Sharing the Bed

Toni was remarkably tolerant about sharing our queen-size bed with a peripatetic cripple. After my first night home, she even said she got a good night's sleep. But as we spent more nights in that bed, I got more active—and she got less sleep.

One morning, about my fifth at home, she jumped out of bed at 6 a.m. and stomped into the bathroom. I recognized the angry stomp of a woman who hasn't slept much. I had got up three or four times that night, and each time I had clunked my path to the bathroom with the walker. I was also not sleeping as well when in the bed, and resorted to performing one of my exercises, the ankle flex, in the middle of the night. It was intended to reduce the chance of blood clotting in the lower leg. I could barely hear the rustle of sheets as I pulled toes up and pushed them down. But I didn't hear well with my hearing aids off at night. Toni, in contrast, was known as "Miss Bat-ears," because she could hear everything. She hadn't mentioned it, but the foot flex had clearly been bothering her.

"It's like Chinese water-torture," she declared over breakfast. "Swish-swish, swish-swish."

"Between that and you getting up at all hours, I can't get much sleep. I'm going to have to go sleep in another bed," she said. "Do you really have to do that exercise in the middle of the night?" she asked

"No, probably not." I was guilty.

Showering with a Bandage

Washing was complicated too. Immersing in a bath was forbidden, for obvious reasons, but showering was okay. I was encouraged to wash in a shower, but told not to wet the bandage over my incision. That sounded difficult.

I had tried practicing a shower before the operation (Toni said I was getting obsessive again), and found it impossible to wash other parts of my body without getting my right thigh wet.

I called the nurses at the hospital, and one told me to tape a plastic bag over the incision and bandage. Aha! Why hadn't they said so?

To be sure, the bandage on the incision was supposed to be waterproof, or at least water resistant. My instructions said it was okay to get a little water on it if you toweled it off promptly. But that seemed a pretty undependable way to protect the bandage.

I went back to basics: a plastic bag and duct tape. I taped the bag to my leg in front of the bandage and across the top and bottom, but I couldn't see and reach around to tape the outer edge. I got Toni to do that. She also found some surgical tape for the purpose, which peeled off without taking as much hair as the duct tape. (Go with surgical tape if you have it.)

I hobbled into our walk-in shower and took a seat on my borrowed shower chair. I sat with my right, replaced, hip farthest from the shower spigots. I enjoyed one big advantage over most showering hip patients—our shower has a sprinkling head on a flexible hose and a small seat-level shelf for soap. (Another patient hung soap and shampoos from strings so he could reach them, but I didn't need to.) I sprayed a stream of warm water over my left side, from head to toe. That felt great!

Turning the water off, I scrubbed with soap and a wash cloth, going from my left to my right, avoiding the taped bag on my right hip. I rinsed the cloth and used that to rinse off parts on my right side that I couldn't safely hit with a stream of water. Finally, bending forward and a little to my left, I used the flexible hose to wash and rinse my hair.

I managed to keep the bandage completely dry. The shower felt great. (Peeling duct tape off did not. I've since learned that Johnson & Johnson sells "Shower Care" bandage protectors, which appear to be designed for this purpose.)

*Guideline Twelve: **Drink lots of fluids***
Drink liquids the day before your surgery to prevent the dehydration that slowed my initial recovery. Also, keep drinking after you go home, to minimize cramping.

*Guideline Thirteen: **Avoid Health Hazards***
If you're overweight, take daily narcotic pain medications (which don't work well for arthritis pain), or smoke or drink alcohol heavily, consider revising your habits. Each of these correlates to higher rates of surgery complications. Some doctors will decline to operate on patients with these conditions.[26]

13

PAIN MANAGEMENT

B efore my surgery, I decided I would use as little anesthesia and narcotic pain medication as possible. I figured my threshold for tolerating pain was pretty high, and opioid abuse was then ravaging my home state of New Hampshire, leaving a trail of overdose deaths, neglected kids and infants born with addiction. Nationally, opioid overdose deaths had tripled in 15 years. I didn't want to join that crowd.

The one Tramadol pill I took my first night home was the last I ever took. My pain level was low, and when I did have some, non-narcotic Tylenol and Naproxen seemed to deal with it.

The hospital had sent me home with 71 tablets of Tramadol, with instructions to take one every four hours, as needed. So I had 70 tablets left over, which seemed like a deplorable waste. More important, it seemed like an invitation to abuse narcotics.

Moschetti told me that the hospital had given me the amount that an average hip or knee replacement patient had required in the past. He maintained that I was very unusual in taking only a single pain pill. Tramadol was the weakest narcotic they prescribed, he said, and I was assigned a low dose rate. That suggested that most patients used much more Tramadol or more-potent narcotics like Oxycodone or Dilaudid.

My interviews didn't suggest I was all that unusual. Almost all the hip replacement patients I interviewed said they took their narcotics for only a day or two.

To be sure, pain is tough to pin down. Lacking any objective pain yardstick, Moschetti noted, doctors rely on patients' evaluations of how much pain they feel and how much narcotic they need to alleviate it. And since drugs work differently on different people, predicting a drug's effectiveness and needed dose is doubly hard.

Opioid drug makers have spent freely to convince doctors that their pills are relatively safe and non-addictive. Some currently face lawsuits claiming they made false and misleading statements.

Frankly, physician convenience and past attitudes may encourage over-prescription. It's easier for doctors to prescribe more pills at one time than to deal with repeated patient requests for more. Doctors also want to get good patient-satisfaction scores, which may affect their compensation. "Overprescribing drugs improves patient satisfaction, but does not improve health," said Brian Sites, my anesthesiologist.

Ten years ago, physicians were criticized for failing to help people relieve pain, which some considered the "5th vital sign." Some said patients should have no pain, even with surgery. This attitude may have contributed to the current opioid epidemic, but it is changing.

Other conditions may have a bearing on sensitivity to pain or vulnerability to addiction. One study co-authored by

Dr. Sites disclosed that individuals with mental disorders used opioids at more than triple the rate of other Americans. The study concluded, "Improving pain management among this population is critical to reduce national dependency on opioids." [27]

Avoiding Dependence

One study found narcotic dependence in 15 to 26 percent of patients who got opioids. Spurred by such findings, the American medical world is looking more skeptically at whether patients need narcotics.[28] A recent study of emergency departments found no significant difference between the short-term pain relief provided by opioids and non-opioid analgesics like ibuprofen (Advil) and acetaminophen (Tylenol).[29] With addiction, as with disease, prevention is easier than treatment. A Journal of the American Medical Association editorial said that substituting non-opioid treatments for pain may prove to be an important step toward reducing opioid addiction.[30]

At DHMC, pain management experts from the anesthesiology department working with the orthopedic surgery department have created a comprehensive approach that offers multiple options for pain management in addition to opioids.

*GUIDELINE FOURTEEN: **Try to Get by With Minimal Narcotics***

I did. So did most of the patients I interviewed. Icing the hip and taking non-steroidal anti-inflammatories can often relieve pain and don't constipate you, as do narcotics. Medicine is moving fast toward using opioids less frequently than in the past, which may reduce addiction.

14

ACHING AND WALKING

Not Supposed to Hurt

David Barlow, my physical therapist, was not impressed when I told him that my hip hurt a lot less than I had expected. "It's not supposed to hurt much," he said.

Still, my sensations evolved. I noticed an ache about five days after surgery. Seven days out of the OR it had grown stronger.

"What's strange is that it goes down my thigh as far as the knee," I said, "far from the spot where I got surgery."

"That's the nerve," said David. "They had to stretch it over to the side to get at the joint." (Moschetti later told me that stretching the muscles may have contributed, too.)

That brought to mind videos and animations that I'd watched, showing surgeons using metal retractors to pull muscles, fascia and other tissues out of their line of sight to the joint. It wasn't hard to imagine a nerve being stretched.

"The aching should go away in another week or two," David said—unless it was badly stretched or cut, in which case it could take much longer. He was right. The ache subsided.

Walking Unaided

A week after my surgery, David got me to walk toward a mirror using one crutch and again, without it. The difference was surprising. I thought I could walk well without the crutch, as long as I took it slowly. What I hadn't realized was that I was tottering. When I stepped onto my right foot I lurched my weight slightly onto that side. I didn't do it when using one crutch, or even a cane.

David explained that my lurch stemmed from a self-protective instinct to avoid straining muscles in the hip. As long as I used something on the opposite side for balance, he said, I wouldn't lurch. He said I should do short stints of walking, but not long ones. "Go ahead and do some laps around your house or walk around a store." I could do it with a crutch, a cane, or without support, he said. "When you get tired, sit down."

He was still urging me to go easy on exercises, and to omit the one that called for me to sit, lift my lower leg and hold the whole leg horizontal for three seconds. My quadriceps had no trouble lifting the lower leg, but it hurt, so I dropped that one.

David had me walking up a few stairs without using my crutches. To my surprise, it didn't hurt, and the right leg seemed strong enough. This was encouraging.

That day, Toni took me out to lunch to celebrate my new hip's first week. We stopped at a flower nursery on the way home and bought geraniums for flower pots. It was refreshing to stroll outside on a warm, sunny day after a week of almost nonstop rain. On our return home, I lugged some feed up to the chicken coop and pulled some weeds from my vegetable patch, without crutches or cane. My hip didn't complain. I murmured, "Thank you, Dr. Moschetti."

15

ONE WEEK OUT: INCISION EXPOSED

Removing the Bandage

Seven days after surgery, I peeled off the bandage over my hip incision, as my loose-leaf binder recommended. Beneath was a 3.75-inch purple line where Moschetti had cut his way in. To one side, I could still make out a trace of the green ink he had used to mark this as the correct hip for surgery. Gone was the blue bruising that had seeped out from under the bandage shortly after surgery.

I became aware that I had some numbness on the side of my thigh, a few inches behind the incision. It seemed to be a consequence of a stretched nerve. I assumed it would come back; if not, I probably wouldn't miss it much. (It did come back months later.)

The area looked almost immaculate. There were no stitches or staples. Instead of slicing the hip, it almost looked like someone had drawn a straight line in purple ink, squiggling the pen a little at the top and bottom. The incision had been sealed shut without stitches. Something was still guarding the surface. As I washed nearby with a cloth, stretching the skin, it reflected crinkled shards of light as if it were coated with plastic wrap. It was glue. My incision was glued shut.

Don't Scrub

I had been told I could get the scar wet in a shower, but not immerse it. (No bath, no hot tub, no swimming.) So, I wondered, should I scrub it with soap or the anti-bacterial cleanser I had used to prep for surgery? I called the hospital. A nurse said I could get it wet in a shower, but added firmly, "do NOT scrub it with ANYTHING."

My directions said to leave the wound open to air or cover it with a light bandage. Nervous about contamination, I taped some non-stick gauze pads over the wound and didn't shower until 24 hours later. Better safe than sorry.

My scar two weeks after surgery

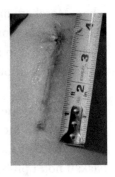

Not very long

PATIENT #5: CAMILLA

SUTURE INFECTION

~

I nfections are rare for hip replacements, but they do happen. Camilla's recovery from hip replacement was "incredibly frustrating." Her incision got infected, and for a month, she had trouble getting the incision to heal.

At the start, Camilla's anterior hip operation seemed to go well. She got out of the hospital the following day and only needed narcotics for pain for about three days. She walked with a cane after about a week.

The problem was that her wound wouldn't fully close. Where her incision had been glued together, three small holes appeared. They gradually expanded, and began oozing puss. Her doctor diagnosed it as a staph infection and scheduled her for surgery that evening.

Seven weeks after the original surgery, the wound was reopened, debrided and flushed to clean out the infection. Surgeons used nylon sutures to sew it back up. Camilla waded into the recovery process again. She received IV antibiotics for two days and was sent home the third day with more antibiotics and a vacuum tube attached to her suture line to capture drainage.

Though her stitches were removed 14 days later, her wound continued to drain from holes that would not stay closed. Almost two months later, Camilla found one more suture emerging next to the incision. After she pulled it out, the holes sealed and her recovery picked up steam. Camilla, it seemed, was allergic to the suture.

In about four months, Camilla felt the hip was almost completely recovered. She played her first game of tennis in years. Soon she was taking short walks, swimming and river kayaking.

Before the onset of hip pain, Camilla had managed to keep and ride a horse. "I could probably ride now," she said nine months after her second operation. "I just don't have the courage yet."

~

16

TRAINING

Getting Off Drugs

A week after surgery, I was still taking two drugs to reduce constipation or soften stool. Belatedly, I realized that these were not necessary, since I was off the narcotic. I stopped taking these drugs and had no negative effects. There was one positive effect: my voice, which had been hoarse for days, returned to normal.

That left me taking aspirin for blood thinning, naproxen for inflammation, and an acid neutralizer to protect the stomach lining from them. If I felt any pain, I took an occasional Tylenol.

Therapy Gets Physical

Nine days after surgery, David started to pick up the pace of my rehabilitation training. He had me **step up** onto an eight-inch platform **and down** off of it, using my right leg to lift and lower my weight. I was surprised that my right leg was significantly weaker than my left. David said that could stem from my favoring that leg before surgery, or just failing to use that leg since the surgery. The strain of my full weight

on my right knee was a little intimidating. David urged me
to not push it.

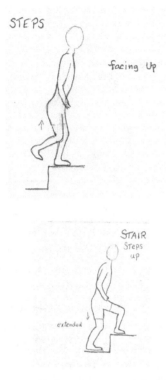

STEPS

facing Up

STAIR
Steps
up

extended

Leg lifts facing up were not too hard.

"YOU'VE GOT a little blood seeping into your lower leg,"
David noted. I twisted to see the back of my right calf. Sure
enough, a shadow of blue spread south of the back of the
knee. Gravity was allowing blood to seep down the back of
my leg from the surgery area. "Don't worry," he said. "It'll be
absorbed by your bloodstream."

David gave me hip **stretching exercises**, some of them

things that I had been unable to do for a year or so due to my arthritis. "If you do these, you'll gain added range of motion" he said. "If you don't, in a month or more your hip will lock in what you have now, and you won't be able to expand your range."

I had a road bike that I could mount on a stand to use it as a stationary bike, but I hadn't used it much because it didn't offer enough resistance.

"You won't want much resistance," said David. Still, he told me to wait another week before trying it. "You're not ready for that yet."

I Drop the Crutches

On my ninth day after surgery, my right thigh was starting to feel almost normal. I walked around the house without crutches or cane. When I walked outside I intended to use a crutch or cane, but often forgot. My goal was to use the leg a fair amount, but not overdo it.

My vegetables and hens benefited from my shortage of other activities. I spent hours weeding my vegetable garden, leaning on my left crutch while scratching out weeds with my right hand. I dropped the crutch and planted rows of spinach and beets, working from my knees. I used one crutch while carrying food and water to our chicken coop.

That evening, friends gave me a lift to the community theater where Toni was performing in the opening night of "Steel Magnolias." The play was delightful; Toni was pleased. But almost two and a half hours on a small, hard seat stretched my hip's tolerance for sitting. After the play, I was so happy to get out of the seat that I walked about 250 yards to the car. I used a cane, but had to walk faster than I wanted to keep up with my friends. When I woke the next morning, pain in my hip said, "Hey stupid, you overdid it yesterday."

My tenth day out, flowers were blooming and my two beehives were abuzz with arriving and departing flights. I spent a few hours assembling more honeycomb frames for my hives. Standing for hours at my work bench didn't bother the hip.

Sitting was more difficult. Later, after I sat reading for an hour or more, I felt stabs of pain when I rose to my feet. Once my hip had got accustomed to the seated position, it got locked in that position. Standing ripped out the locking restraints. Fortunately, the hip loosened up quickly, and felt comfortable once I took a few steps.

By then I was beginning to shower almost normally. I pushed the shower seat out of the way and washed myself standing. Though I tried to minimize water running over the scar, it did get wet as I scrubbed that side of my upper body and shampooed my hair. I stuck with nurses' orders not to scrub the actual incision area, and when drying myself, I was careful not to rub it with the towel.

17

PAIN & PARANOIA

Pain Growing

Twelve days out of the operating room, I got worried. The pains in my right hip were growing, instead of fading, and I didn't know why. My main concern was that I hurt when I first rose to a standing position and began walking. I felt the following:

- soreness down the front of my thigh from hip to knee.
- sharp pains in or near the joint, and,
- stiffness and soreness along the incision.

To be sure, the pain level remained fairly low—I figured maybe 2 to 3 on a 10-point scale—and it usually eased as I moved around and limbered up. But I worried that it hit more areas, not less, and that it seemed to be growing more, rather than less, intense.

Maybe the exercises were causing the pain. David's stair-steps up and down were the first non-wimpy exercises I had tried. I thought they could explain my rising quad pain, but probably not the others.

David had also assigned me some more modest **stretching** exercises, including one that twisted both legs and hip to the left side. I could feel that pulling on something behind the right hip joint.

Perhaps I was walking around too much on that leg. I asked, "How do you know when you're doing too much?"

"When it hurts," David replied.

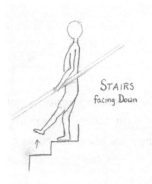

STAIRS
facing Down

I backed off a bit on the stair-stepping workouts, supporting more of my weight on my arms. That seemed to help. I dismissed the changes as growing pains. Despite the new complaints, my general mobility seemed to be still improving.

Tick Fears

On my thirteenth day out of surgery, I found my first tick. The discovery came about 5:30 a.m. Light was starting to filter in our windows and I was accepting wakefulness as irreversible. I felt a point of irritation on my right side about eight inches above and a little behind the hip. Feeling for it with my hand in bed, I thought it might be an insect bite.

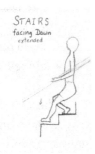

STAIRS
facing Down
extended

Lowering a leg facing down was the hard part.

I gave up on sleep and examined my right side in the bathroom mirror. Instead of a tiny red bug bite, I saw a distinct dark spot. I managed to squeeze tweezers over the spot. Examining the tweezers, I found a tiny black body with wiggling legs: a very small tick. I washed it down the sink and showered, using antibacterial soap on the tick bite.

A small rash reddened around the dark bite mark, but failed to produce the bullseye rash that I had come to associate with Lyme disease. I had no flu-like symptoms, but the hospital's warnings against infection had made me hyper-vigilant. I couldn't take a bath for six weeks. I'd have to get antibiotics just to get my teeth cleaned in the next two months. So I asked the orthopaedics department whether I should get antibiotics for the risk of Lyme disease. The nurses seemed unconcerned. They referred me to my personal physician. I had an appointment for an annual checkup in a few weeks; I figured I'd mention it to her then. (I didn't, and survived.)

GUIDELINE FIFTEEN: **If Workouts Hurt, Cut Back**

Expect some pain as you exercise and start to heal. When pain mounts, do less.

TWO WEEKS OUT: STRETCH, WORK, DRIVE

A bout two weeks after surgery, my physical therapist introduced a set of **stretches:** leaning against a counter and angling the hip toward it (IT band and abductor muscle), squatting back on my haunches to push my knee toward my chest (quadriceps), lying on my back and pulling my knee toward my chest while trying to straighten the leg (hamstrings).

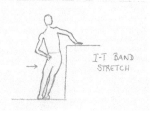

I-T BAND STRETCH

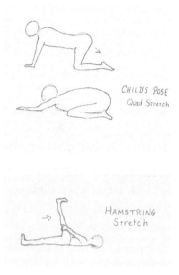

CHILD'S POSE
Quad Stretch

HAMSTRING
Stretch

He also added to my **strengthening workouts:** lying on my back and pushing my hips up (gluteus maximus), and more stepping up or down a stair-step (quadriceps).

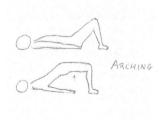

ARCHING

The exercises seemed to continue my progress toward doing light work. I spent half of one day moving a mulch pile off our driveway, shoveling it into a lawn trailer and making a pile in the woods. I cleaned out our garage, sweeping and mopping. For work around home I walked without pain.

It occurred to me that I might be ready to take Nell and Piper for a short walk, but after the first 100 yards, I turned back. The longer I walked, the more I felt pains in my hip muscles. I wasn't sure I should do more, so I didn't.

Driving

I hadn't left home for two weeks without Toni as my driver. We were both getting a little tired of my relying on her as my chauffeur. My binder said no driving for four-to-six weeks, until my surgeon approved it.

I encountered an orthopaedic surgeon from New York who supported the idea of not driving. "It's not just the drugs," he said. "There have been studies that showed that reaction time of the muscles take about a month to recover."

Two weeks out of surgery, I called the hospital and a nurse rejected my suggestion that I resume driving. I figured that was a knee-jerk response. She cited the slow reactions of people on narcotics, so she clearly had not factored into her response that I was not taking narcotics. I had driven my lawn tractor with no problems. I figured that I'd stay off the roads for a few more days, but that the time was approaching to climb back behind the steering wheel.

Almost three weeks out of surgery, at Toni's urging, I drove myself to physical therapy. It seemed like a good test. The PT office was about 4 miles up a lightly-traveled highway. I wouldn't need quick reactions.

I drove myself. As best I could tell, driving at that point was no problem for me. Later, I found some studies suggesting I could have resumed driving even sooner.

GUIDELINE SIXTEEN: *Be Skeptical of the Warnings against Driving*

Some physicians call for patients to wait four or six weeks after right hip replacement before driving. This may be driven as much by liability concerns as research. Discomfort in the hip can make driving uncomfortable for a week or two, especially for replaced right hips. But while narcotics impair reactions, most patients are off drugs in less than a week. And while hip surgery has been shown to slow muscle reaction temporarily, studies differ on how long that's a problem. Some studies suggest normal reaction speed returns within two-to-four weeks, others say as little as two days.[31,32,33,34]

PATIENT #6: JEANIE

"I AM NOT A WIMP"

~

Jeanie proved hip replacement patients don't have to be immobile. Her husband, Buzz, drove her across Florida two days after her surgery, and 1,500 miles two weeks later. She was driving herself in two or three weeks, she says, and after a month she felt as if she could do almost anything.

Jeanie's arthritis had come on fast. Over three months, the 70-year-old recalls, she progressed from feeling no hip pain in her right hip to feeling pain so great that, "I was barely able to walk."

At first, doctors said her hip x-rays didn't look bad enough for surgery. She tried steroid shots and physical therapy. She joined a "spinning" class to keep in shape. The pain grew progressively worse; so much so, she quit spinning.

She went back to a doctor, saying, "I am not a wimp. I have a high pain threshold," but there's something seriously wrong with my hip. After another round of x-rays, the doctor agreed, and scheduled anterior hip replacement.

After general anesthesia wore off, she was able to walk later that day and leave the hospital the next. Her medical team asked her to stay one more night in case complications arose—in a neighboring hotel; not the hospital, she says, because of its infection risk.

When Buzz drove her three hours to their winter home on Florida's west coast the second day out of surgery, they stopped about once an hour so she could climb out and shuffle about with a walker. She did exercises to rebuild muscles in her hip. After she used a walker for about a week, she went without any support. She said she couldn't get comfortable with a cane.

Two weeks after surgery, her Florida doctors cleared her for the drive north to New Hampshire. Buzz drove, and they took their time, driving about four or five hours per day. Though doctors warned her not to drive for four to six weeks, she felt confident she could drive sooner, and did.

In the next few months, Jeanie tended gardens, rode a horse and a bike and played golf. Less than a year after surgery she and Buzz rode bikes from Stockholm to Copenhagen, logging 30-50 miles per day. She concedes their "ebikes" supplied electric battery boosts for hills. But she called that a concession to age rather than hips; they had to keep up with their children and grandchildren. Even with the boost, she recalls, pain occasionally stabbed the repaired hip. "I probably pushed myself too far," she says. Doctors told her the pain was normal.

She emerged an advocate for hip replacement. "Don't dread the operation," she advises hip sufferers. "Do what you have to do. You're going to change your life."

"If I had to have the other hip done, I'd have no hesita-
tion at all." she says. "I'm 100 percent happy with my
surgery."

~

THREE WEEKS OUT

More Exercises

It was time to ramp up physical therapy. On the three-week anniversary of my surgery, I told David, "The hip seems to be recovering well, but I am alarmed that my right leg is a lot weaker than my left."

"Your progress is completely normal," he said, "including the weakness."

What worried me was that it was a real effort for my right knee to support my body weight while I lowered my left foot one stair-step, facing down, and raised it back up. David's instructions the previous week had been to do this 15 times a set and repeat two more sets each day. He also called for stepping forward, up and back down, 15 times, three times a day. Stepping up wasn't too hard. But my right knee strained when I stepped down. I could get through one set of 15, but fearing damage, I needed to rest the knee before I tried another.

Okay, said David, do eight of the step downs, or don't step down all the way. I could work my way up to 15.

David added two **balance exercises**: standing on a foam

pillow on one foot; and standing with one foot on the floor and bending forward at the waist.

He also prescribed new **strength builders:**

- squatting and stepping sideways with a blue band around my thighs, rising to full height at the end of each side-step;
- pushing out one leg to the side, then the other, against resistance of the blue band;
- pulling one leg backward, then the other, against the blue band.
- lifting my knee above waist-level 15 times, first with one leg, then the other;
- lunge forward onto one knee, dropping the other knee close to the ground.

ELASTIC BAND PULLS

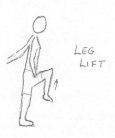

LEG
LIFT

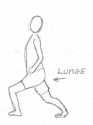

LUNGE

He encouraged me to ride a stationary bike. When I got home, I mounted my road bike on the stand that made it a stationary exerciser. It worked.

At home, I faced unanimous demand that I start **walking** more: when I approached the mud room door Nell licked me and Piper jumped and spun. This was border collie for, "Isn't it time for a hike?" Toni had been doing the dog-walking chores, and was clearly ready for me to begin picking up my share.

In fact, walking was becoming easier. David encouraged me to walk for 15 or 20 minutes at a time, but avoid steep or uneven ground. That ruled out the forested trails behind our house. But it left open other options.

One day I walked the quarter-mile down to our mail box and back. That called for negotiating a fairly steep hill, which, David said, was not good for my hip on the descent. It also was a bit short for my crazy border collies. So I figured out where I could take the dogs for a level hike. I drove them about three miles away to where we could walk along River Road, which was not only flat but closed to through traffic. The border collies were thrilled. I walked, trying not to totter. Nelly and Piper ran in and out of the woods and the river. A good time was had by all.

Snap the IT Band

I was walking with almost no pain. The occasional ache in my right quad had almost disappeared, but I had not returned to normal. I sometimes felt pain when I rose from a sitting position and started to walk. It quickly went away when I started moving around, especially if I gave it a second to adjust to a standing and walking position. Still, I found it hard to settle into a normal walking gait. I felt myself unconsciously protecting the right leg, sometimes hopping from the left leg, as I had before the operation.

Also, something was snapping in my hip joint every time I stepped upward or down on the right leg. It felt like a rubber band was stretching around my joint, then sliding off it with a snap as the hip straightened up. Was there something wrong with the way the joint was assembled? I'd heard there are sometimes follow-up "revision" surgeries to fix things that weren't right. I hoped I wouldn't need one. That would kill my kayaking trip and delay resumption of normal life.

"That's the IT band," said David. The band runs down the outside of the thigh from the pelvis down to the knee. David had me lean against a kitchen counter with the right hip angled in toward it. It just needed to stretch some, he said.

GEAR—WHAT Was Useful?

As I approached my hip's four-week anniversary, I returned all my borrowed surgery support stuff—the shower seat, walker, crutches and cane. I had used the walker for the first week, the seat for the first ten days, and the crutches and cane at times for most of the month.

Most of the other gear was helpful, but not necessary. I used the:

- sock puller for a couple of weeks, until I could reach my toes;
- leg-lifter for a couple of weeks, never to be used again;
- long shoe horn for most of the month, and is nice to have later;
- long-handled sponge once or twice—largely a shower ornament;
- long "grabber" never, except as a toy for my three-year-old grandson.

20

FOUR WEEKS OUT: WALK, CHIP AND PUTT

The day after my fourth-week anniversary, I took Nell and Piper for a longer walk. Wielding walking sticks, I trudged down my driveway and along our little road. About a half-mile from our door, we turned into one of the well-traveled forest paths. After crossing a bridge over a brook, the footpath headed uphill at moderate steepness, leaf litter alternating with muddy patches. At an intersection of paths, I turned left and walked to one side, toward the stream. I walked slowly, and tried to keep using the sticks.

The dogs were nowhere to be seen. I whistled and called. No response. I feared they had been so disgusted with my snail's pace that they had left me. But they were working dogs, and stayed on the job. First Piper came charging down the trail, then Nelly. Each black and white flash ran up to greet me, putting on the brakes a few feet away from my legs. Having checked in, they pivoted and ran ahead again, full speed.

When I reached the stream crossing, they were ranging along the opposite side, where the trail ahead climbed steeply uphill. I didn't want to push my hip that hard yet, so I headed back, calling the collies. They raced past. I trudged carefully back to our house.

My hike that day amounted to about 1.5 miles. I felt no pain.

(Miniature) Golf

About the same time, I started to practice my chipping and putting on the local golf course. I didn't try swinging longer clubs yet. I hoped that would start soon, but I was waiting for doctor's orders.

Dr. Moschetti told me about one patient who came in for his one-month post-operative checkup saying he had just played 18 holes of golf.

"I hope you took a cart," said Moschetti.

"Nope," said the patient. "I walked and carried my clubs."

"That was not a good idea," Moschetti told me. "We want to make sure that the bone has had a chance to grow into the porous surface" of the replacement parts that had been installed in the hip. The stability and longevity of the parts depended on a good bond. Too much strain, too early, could cause problems.

For two days, I spent an hour or two working on my short game with ten golf balls. I was lousy—no surprise. Maybe the enforced focus on chipping and putting would pay more dividends than my usual push to hit a driver and long irons. More important, I was still pain-free.

Weakness Lingers

The main symptom that still worried me was weakness. I still found it hard to lower my left leg, while bending my right knee, until the left heel touched the next stair down. I was doing sets of 10, rather than the prescribed 15, and not always going all the way down.

David had me sit on a low seat and rise to a standing position with all my weight on one leg. I could do it with my left leg, but not my right.

I was going to have to build up my right leg. But I came to the view that I shouldn't push it too hard yet. Doing so, I feared, might damage my right knee. David said I was still in the healing phase, and shouldn't push hard on any exercise for another couple of weeks.

The previous week I had gone to the gym and tried out a few of the workout machines set at low resistance levels. I had squeezed thighs together and pushed them outwards. I curled my hamstrings, lifted my lower leg forward using my quadriceps, and rode a stationary bike. I didn't do anything that called for straining. The workout felt good. David said I could do more, but keep the resistance light.

21

"ANYTHING YOU FEEL COMFORTABLE DOING"

After Four Weeks, the Light Turns Green
Going back to the hospital for a hip check, I felt like a student on the eve of graduation. In the x-ray department, a technician shot pictures of my hips and pelvis. After an associate looked at my scar, I met Moschetti.

"So," he announced as he took a seat, "how are you feeling?"

"Great!" I said, "thanks to you."

He showed an x-ray. My pelvis and femurs showed up as faint white shadows on a gray background. On one side, a bright-white shadow of metal appeared: the semi-circle of the socket in my pelvis and the ball connected to the tapered stem that stuck into my femur. It had become a familiar image in books and Web sites, but I had a hard time believing that the hardware I was looking at was in my own right hip.

He asked if I felt any difference in the length of my legs. I hadn't.

Using a computer mouse, he drew a straight line on the screen across the base of my pelvis from one leg to the other.

"See, the line goes to about the middle of this little bump, the lesser trochanter, on each leg. They look about even."

That's how I knew that my general practitioner's nurse had misread my height. At my annual physical, she measured my height as 6 feet and 0.44 inches. I wondered if Moschetti had lengthened one leg. The answer was no; I was still just shy of six feet.

Moschetti explained that prior to surgery he had uploaded my x-ray into a computer templating software program, which helped him pick the right sized parts to make the legs about the same length. He had checked the parts again in the body with x-rays in the operating room, and he had various sizes available in case the planned pieces didn't look right.

All of this was interesting, but soon I got to the point. "When can I go out and play golf or ride my bike?"

"You can do anything you feel comfortable doing," he said.

My throat choked back the "Wahoo!" that my brain was yelling. I asked about working out with weights or resistance. I asked about climbing mountains. The answer didn't change. "Anything you feel comfortable..."

I drove home, had lunch, and collected my golf bag and shoes. I hit a few lobs onto a practice green, drove to the golf shop, rented a cart and headed onto the course.

Real Golf

It was a cool June day. Sun alternated with clouds. Recent rains had kept the grass lush and green. To my surprise, it didn't hurt my hip to swing a driver. My right hip had to turn, but that didn't seem to bother it. As a right-handed golfer, most swing stress pushed onto the left hip. I also tried to swing easily.

I told the golf shop I might not play 18; I'd see how it

went. It went well. I didn't always hit the ball well, but I had no pain. I took my time. I played 18, and was just glad to be out there.

That night, I sent my favorite golf partners a note: "I'm back!"

GUIDELINE SEVENTEEN: **Get Outside**

As soon as you're cleared by your medical team, enjoy light exercise.

PATIENT #7: AMOS

MAKING LEGS EQUAL

~

Amos's hip replacements were due to injuries as well as osteoarthritis.

Osteoarthritic hip pain developed in Amos's 60s after he slammed one hip onto an icy ski slope. When it hurt so bad he couldn't ski, he sought medical advice.

Doctors had news for Amos: one leg was a full inch longer than the other—apparently from faulty repairs of both legs that he broke in high school.

Amos had pushed his unequal legs for decades. Aside from skiing and playing competitive singles tennis, he had run 18 marathons. Along the way, he had had surgeries to repair both of his Achilles tendons and one knee. Amos was a glutton for punishment.

Orthopaedic surgeons replaced his hip and equalized his leg lengths. He had to re-learn to walk on equally long legs, but the new hip worked well. A few years after his original hip replacement, the other one gave him trouble. After cortisone shots failed to help, he got that one done, too.

Amos says he got what he wanted from hip implants. He still plays tennis and skis. He did have to give up running. Instead, he says, "I bike a lot."

∾

22

SEX

One other activity I felt comfortable doing was having sex.

When I first got back from surgery full intimacy was out of the question. I was using a leg-lifting strap to get in bed.

One review of the medical literature concluded that hip replacements improved sexual activity for many patients.[35] I saw some illustrations of what positions were safe for hip-replacement patients to use when starting their recovery, with different guidance for males and females.

I never needed the coaching. By one month's time, my hip felt secure. I didn't worry about positions. My wife and I resumed intimacy. She was more worried about my hip than I was.

23

FIVE TO SEVEN WEEKS: ON TRAIL, IN RIVER

A s my five-week anniversary passed, I was back on the trails with Piper and Nelly. Which was a good thing, since Toni had left for a horse show in Massachusetts. I started by doing our once-standard two-mile hike—uphill through forest and a hay field to a lateral trail across the shoulder of the hill and down into a valley and a 20-foot-wide brook. Piper and Nell raced through the tall grass, charged through the trees and lay in the brook to cool off. I used walking sticks and trod slower than usual. My trainer, David, had cautioned against hard heel strikes on the downhill paths. I took mincing steps to avoid them.

To my delight, I was pain free. I didn't feel secure jumping or running, but walking or biking were no problem. A few days later I took the dogs to the Lyme Hill Conservation Area. We climbed up one hill and then down a forested path to Grant's Brook. The round trip was about three miles, with lots of up and down. My right leg was tired at the end, but my hip felt good.

David was surprised that Moschetti had given me a green light to do "anything I felt comfortable doing." The therapist recalled the days when hip replacement patients didn't even start rehab work until four to six weeks after surgery. He confessed he didn't have a lot of additional exercises for me.

Six Weeks: Off Drugs and On to Fishing

At the end of my fifth week out of surgery, I went trout fishing in the headwaters of the Connecticut River in the northern tip of New Hampshire. Donning hip waders and carrying my fly rod, I wondered if this was going to prove too much for the new hip. The river floor was rocky and water rushing over it varied from six inches to more than three feet deep. Six inches, no problem; three feet, the force of the water constantly threatened to push me downstream. Rocks were slippery and unstable. One misstep and I was going swimming. I broke off a thick stick to use for a balance, and waded in.

In two days of exploring the river, I caught a few nice fish and gave my hip a good workout. Stepping against the current across and upstream was like pushing against resistance machines at the gym, only better. The water pressure was strong but flexible. I stumbled and fell into the water once, but my hip made no complaint.

After I reached the six-week mark, I ran out of anti-inflammatory Naproxen. I had quit the aspirin about ten days earlier. Without the naproxen, my hip gave me little twinges that I had not been feeling, but these abated as my muscles and limbs warmed up. I played my third round of golf, this time with a cart, the same day I trekked with the dogs to the top of Lyme Hill (1.8 miles, a lot of it vertical). I felt uncomfortable only when I stood after sitting for more than ten minutes.

Seven Weeks: Bridge-Building

The next week I joined a bridge-building crew. A

neighbor and a group from the local conservation commission had staged building materials next to the brook I crossed daily with my dogs. I had to pick my way across stones or fallen logs, because the bridge that once spanned it was gone. This group set out to build a new one.

Our first task was to haul three 35-foot hemlock logs across the chasm and anchor them on each end. The hemlock was heavy. It took at least six of us to lift one end. We used a cable and hoist to slide the logs across the stream, but first we had to manually lift and drag the logs into position.

I stepped up and grabbed one of the loops of webbing to lift and pull.

"Bend your knees, not your backs," said one of the crew leaders. "One, two, three, heave."

We slid the timber a few inches at a time. We had all but finished moving the first log before it dawned on me that I was crazy to put that much weight on my new hip. I had a flash of terror about driving my stem down hard enough to split my femur. I promptly surrendered my spot lifting heavy objects, and looked for things I could do with my cordless drill and hammer. Miraculously, I hadn't damaged the joint.

GUIDELINE EIGHTEEN: Avoid Stressing the New Hip

Jumping, running, lifting heavy objects, and falling are good to avoid after surgery. They could put heavy stress on your new hip.

NAPPING

Though feeling good, I often ran out of energy in the middle of the day. When that happened, I sat down, picked up a magazine and promptly fell sound asleep. This was less a restful nap than the sleep of the living dead. Energy drained from me in a rush. It wasn't like I chose to take a nap. It was more like the need to sleep overwhelmed me. An hour or 90 minutes seemed to be enough. I would return to the land of the living.

These power failures happened for a couple of months after the surgery. Friends in their 70s said this wasn't unusual. "I like to take naps," said one college friend. "You shouldn't feel that taking a nap is a sign of weakness."

I found it worrisome. Before surgery I had taken a midday nap on rare occasions. But in the first month after surgery it happened almost every day, and it seemed to flow from sheer exhaustion. Moschetti told me this was "pretty common after hip surgery." Fortunately, the power failures became less frequent in the second month and continued to fade over time.

EIGHT WEEKS: HIKE A SMALL MOUNTAIN

About two months after surgery, our friend Vic suggested we hike up Mount Cardigan, one of the smaller and more easily accessible peaks in New Hampshire. Vic, who worked for the Vermont State Parks as a young man, had led Toni and me on four or five hikes in the mountains of New Hampshire and Vermont. This time he was eager to do something relatively easy to test out a troublesome knee, which dovetailed perfectly with my desire to test my hip.

Our wives joined us. I carried two lunches and water in a backpack and wielded walking sticks. As we headed out on the trail, my hip felt fine. Would that last?

The trail up Cardigan was rocky and steep in places. It rose 1,220 ft. through forest to a largely bald granite top, capped with a fire-spotter's tower. The climb probably took us about two hours, so it was after 3 p.m. when we found seats on the granite top, broke out lunch and watched graceful wind turbines turning in distant forested mountains.

The mid-summer weather gods rewarded us. It was cool

and sunny, with light breezes. I felt comfortable in a long-sleeved tee-shirt. On the way down, my right hip was still feeling fine. I was tired, but the right leg didn't seem any worse than the left. And while I continued to try to find soft landings for my right heel, the downhill heel strike no longer seemed jarring. The joint and its muscles seemed more robust.

PATIENT #8: ROSEANNE

BATTLING ADVERSITY

~

Recovering from hip replacement surgery can be a long, tough, haul. –Just ask Roseanne.

"Everyone is different," my doctors told me. Most of the hip replacement patients profiled in this book recovered most of their strength and mobility in a month or two. Not everyone can do that.

Seven months after her total hip replacement, Roseanne was still limping. The (abductor) muscle on the back and outside of her new left hip was still sore and weak. She lurched over that leg as she walked, and was still using a cane.

An array of other health problems had impeded Roseanne's recovery from surgery:

- a long-damaged right knee limited the physical therapy she could do;
- she was told extra weight in her belly could increase her risk that an anterior incision might

get infected, so she chose to undergo posterior surgery;

- having only one kidney, she was reluctant to take anti-inflammatories like ibuprofen, which can cause kidney damage in sensitive persons;
- without anti-inflammatories, she relied more heavily on pain pills, and;
- gastrointestinal illnesses laid her low twice, interrupting recovery.

Roseanne puts it this way: "My complications are like, complicated."

She primarily blames the stomach illnesses for impeding her recovery. "That really set me back," she recalls. Each time, "I ended up in bed, sick for a week, not doing PT, not exercising."

A high school teacher, Roseanne got her hip replaced in April and took the spring and summer off. She figured she would walk normally into class five months later to start the fall semester. Instead, she hobbled with a cane from class to class. She needed the cane to get in and out of her low-slung car.

Feeling she had made little progress, she returned to physical therapy. Slowly, she built strength. In December, eight months after surgery, she finally dropped the cane. She walked more, but the knee limited how much she could do.

Like Neil, the avid hiker, she faced a new question: should I fix the knee?

⪡

26

NINE WEEKS: BIKING HILLS

I was feeling pretty confident of my hip's recovery by nine weeks. I played another round of golf with some young guys, taking carts. I mowed our lawn, harvested beets from my maturing vegetable garden, and took my first bike ride to Lyme and back.

I had ridden along River Road a few weeks earlier, which might have totaled ten miles. But I had chosen that route to avoid hills. I had walked up one long hill to get back to my house.

This time I tackled hills. Lyme is only five miles away. I had to climb one hill to get to the highest point on Lyme Road. From there I could ride down three long hills, separated by flat portions, to reach the little town (a classic New England town with a steepled Congregational church and rectangular "green"). Going up the first hill, I noticed a muscle in my groin was hurting a little, so I slowed a bit. I soon realized it was my left groin that was bothering me, not the right leg with the new hip, so I ignored it and the pain went away. On my return, I had to climb those three hills. Both legs felt fine. In fact, I couldn't tell which leg was recovering from surgery. They seemed equal in strength and comfort.

No Jumping

There were still things I was not trying. I was not running, jumping, or kicking my legs high, Rockette-style. (Toni noted I hadn't been much of a Rockette, ever.) But I did kick legs over a three-foot moveable fence we were using to keep our free-ranging chickens from digging up Toni's flower gardens. That felt okay.

I had one last appointment with David, my physical therapist. I told him the leg was coming along well. He seemed surprised that it had responded so quickly. David certified my hip therapy as complete.

TWELVE WEEKS: KAYAKING WITH ORCAS

A t last, I arrived at the big challenge I had anticipated months before. Toni and I met Grant in Seattle. Together with our friend Warren, we drove north through Vancouver Island to go sea kayaking where orcas, better known as killer whales, are known to hang out.

I had yet to find any hidden weakness in my right hip. The most common pain I had felt in my hips had come when I stood up after sitting for more than a few minutes. So, kayaks presented a new challenge. I figured long periods sitting and paddling could cause problems. Also, paddling a small craft in open water left little opportunity for moving the leg around.

I didn't need to worry; the hip did fine. We usually paddled for less than two hours at a time. We saw lots of orcas; some even surfaced between our kayaks. We also saw a bear, an eagle, seals and dolphins. Sleeping bags on cots proved comfortable enough. It was a great trip. We agreed this wasn't roughing it. Even the Canadian border agent had the new word for it: we were "glamping." (luxury camping)

GOLF IMPROVES

For years, my golf game had been terrible. I was convinced that I could get back to shooting in the 80s, as I had in my youth, if I just played often enough. But when I first started playing regularly in retirement I had trouble keeping my scores from soaring above 100.

The first outings after my surgery, I posted scores in the mid-90s, which I felt pretty good about. I hadn't been able to play for months, so I assumed those scores would come down.

Running was no longer a good idea for me, and I had given up tennis decades ago, so I focused on golf for a few months. I was still erratic, but the scores in the 80s came occasionally. I even got my first hole in one.

Was better golf due to the surgery? I doubted it. I figured I improved by playing more and relaxing. But who knows? One study of professional golfers who had arthroscopic hip surgeries (not necessarily total joint replacements) showed they improved the length of their drives, though not the frequency of hitting greens in regulation.[36]

PATIENT # 9: RITCHIE

GOLF IN THE 80S

~

Ritchie loved playing golf so much, it nearly killed him. But dedication and a hip replacement put him back on the links.

At 86 years of age, my beloved uncle Ritchie flipped a golf cart into a sand trap. The cart rolled over him and broke his femur. That would have ended the golf career of a less ardent duffer, but not Ritchie. He got a titanium rod inserted into his left leg and six months later he played in a golf tournament.

Then the rod came loose. He stopped playing golf. "It was pretty damned painful," he recalls. "I was on a walker. I couldn't even lie on my back without it hurting."

Ten months after the original surgery, Ritchie was back on the operating room table. Doctors "took everything out and started fresh," he says. They put in a new rod and replaced his hip joint.

Ritchie spent four nights in the hospital and another four in a rehabilitation unit, but the result was good. A couple of days after surgery, he stopped taking Oxycodone; and he says, "I haven't had any pain ever since."

Ritchie did have to go back for a staph infection—doctors reopened the wound, flushed it out and put him on intravenous antibiotics—but the wound healed "pretty quickly."

Getting back on the links was not so quick. After months of inactivity, Ritchie's leg muscles had atrophied. He used a walker for about a month and went through about three months of physical therapy (his second round). He was driving after two months, chipping and putting in about three months and finally, after nine months, playing 18 holes of golf again.

Ritchie accepted that he couldn't hit the long ball. For a guy who was used to scoring in the 70s, it was hard to accept scoring over 100. But he kept at it. Before long, he was shooting his age.

"At 88 years old, I'm damned lucky to be out on the golf course," he says. "It's been such fun for me, playing that game."

∽

29

SIXTEEN WEEKS: A SERIOUS MOUNTAIN

I n late September, I decided to put the new hip to a test: Mt. Moosilauke. This mountain rises east of the Connecticut River Valley to a height of 4,802 ft. above sea level, almost 3,300 ft. above the trail head I used. The 7.8 mi. round trip would take about seven hours, including about an hour for lunch on top.

I thought my hip was ready for this, but I wasn't sure. Since Toni and I had just signed up for a major hike in Patagonia five months away. I wanted to see how far I could push my new hip—and the other one, too.

Vic Henningsen graciously agreed to join me. He was still testing that wobbly knee. We parked at 9:30 on a surprisingly cool morning and headed east, with Nelly and Piper leading. Within minutes we joined the Appalachian Trail. It ascended gently through mixed conifer and hardwood forest, then ramped up, turning increasingly rocky and steep. Whoever laid out this trail, like most of the Appalachian Trail, had no interest in switchbacks. Trail crews had built occasional stone steps. Aside from those, we picked our way up through boulders and webs of roots left hanging in air by soil erosion. As we ascended we left behind deciduous trees and the conifers shrank in height. I started wondering if we were off the trail. Around noon we emerged onto a gentler "carriage road," that signaled we had it made. Almost a mile across a saddle of short firs took us to the bald, windblown summit.

We enjoyed clear views in all directions. Crows glided on the wind rising up the west slope. The Connecticut River meandered in the west, with Vermont's Green Mountains rising beyond it. The Presidential Range lined the northeastern horizon. Taking refuge from a chilling wind in the ruins of a stone shelter, we ate lunch. My legs were tired, but I felt no aches or pains.

Overstepping?

Marching down was another story. About halfway down, a sharp pain stabbed my right hip. The pain returned on a smaller scale from time to time. I couldn't put my finger on what was causing it, but I knew the complaints came from the joint I had replaced. I slowed my pace and tried to make sure I didn't come down hard on that right leg.

On lower slopes, the stones thinned out and the steepness eased, but my legs started getting wobbly. I found myself leaning back slightly as I stepped forward and downhill.

I worried about that sharp pain. Did that mean my cup had shifted in its socket? Could the stem in my femur have moved?

I didn't know, but whatever it was didn't get worse. By treading carefully on it I was able to get back to the car, trailing Vic and the dogs for the last mile.

I drove back to where Vic had parked, then headed home for a shower and a dinner date. My legs were pretty worn out, but I didn't fall asleep in my soup. The next day I took the dogs on a two-mile hike in the afternoon. No pain. The hike had approached the limit that my legs could tolerate; but as long as that sharp pain didn't return, I counted it as a successful test of new equipment.

WHO GETS HIP REPLACEMENTS?

Close to 10 percent of the U.S. residents over 18 suffer from OA, which causes more than 90 percent of hip replacements.[37,38] This has included slightly more women than men and a growing share of middle-aged persons. Though the disease crops up mostly in older persons, middle-aged OA sufferers aged 45-64, got 42 percent of total hip replacements in 2012, up from only 27 percent in 1997.[39,40]

After surgery, most hip replacement patients have gone to a rehabilitation facility before returning home, but that is changing. In 2012, one study found almost 40 percent of such patients went home from the hospital, more than double the share that did so in 1997.[41] Of the 11 patients I interviewed, mostly family and friends, only one went to a rehab residential facility, and that was my uncle Rich, then 86 years old, who was enduring his second round of surgery for a broken femur. All the others went home, mostly after one night in a hospital.

That's increasingly typical. As medical facilities improve

surgical techniques and reduce anesthesia and narcotic use, hip replacement patients are leaving hospitals sooner. One study found the mean length of stay dropped to 3.2 days in 2012, down from 4.9 days in 1997.[42] Some facilities are releasing selected patients home on the day of surgery.

Complications

"Complications" is a polite medical term for something going wrong. Dislocation is the most frequent complication for hip surgeries, followed by mechanical loosening of components where they were attached to the pelvis or femur. Infection, pulmonary embolism, cracked femur, heart attack and stroke are potential complications, but each occurs in less than 1 percent of cases. Curiously, smokers and obese patients prove to be much more likely to suffer from infection of the surgical space. Adverse reactions to metal debris, or "metallosis", have been a problem with some metal-on-metal joints, both in hip resurfacings and replacements. They can cause a wide range of symptoms from fatigue and formation of soft tissue masses called pseudotumors to dissolution of muscle and bone. And women prove to be more sensitive than men to the metal fragments. Still, many metal-on-metal joints seem to work fine.

Orthopedists use another curious word for situations where a hip replacement isn't working properly and must be redone. They call it a "revision." That sounds like a simple exchange of one thing with another, but it's not that simple. Basically, a doctor has to repeat the original operation, extract the defective parts and put in new ones. So the patient faces a whole new recovery process. And worse, revision patients' mean length of stay has been longer, over 5 days, and the cost almost double that of original hip replacements. The risk of "revision" is significant. One study found it was 2 percent risk the first year, rising about 1 percent per year for the next 12, so the total risk gets into the mid-teens.

31

DENTAL CLEANING CLEARED

Warnings about the risk of post-surgical dental work were rapidly changing. The binder that I got from DHMC before surgery said I needed to "take antibiotics prior to *any* dental procedures for the life of your joint replacement."

That had been a standard warning for many years. The concern focused on bacteria that could enter your bloodstream from cuts in your gums. Doctors worried that these could infect joint implants or the disturbed tissues around them. An infection could require more surgery and heavy doses of antibiotics.

But the medical community was moving away from prophylactic use of antibiotics. The American Academy of Orthopaedic Surgeons found no evidence that dental work was causing infections, or that taking antibiotics before oral care can help prevent them.

At my pre-surgical briefing, I was told not to have dental work for two weeks before or six months after my hip surgery. Thereafter, I was supposed to decide whether to take antibiotics based on a risk-benefit analysis in consultation with my doctor.

The risks were said to be greater for patients with compromised immune systems. Prophylactic antibiotics were suggested for patients with diabetes, rheumatoid arthritis, cancer, or steroid users.

I didn't fit in any of these categories. Moschetti said I didn't need antibiotics before dental work, so about six months after my surgery I got my teeth cleaned without drugs, and I survived.

PATIENT #10: ERIC

BOUNCING BACK

≈

E ric put my recovery to shame. He started hiking after one week and walked up a small mountain after two. He danced away the night after four weeks and kite-boarded after six.

To be sure, he had youth going for him. Only 30 when he had his hips done, he was half the age of the typical hip replacement patient. On the other hand, he had *both* hip joints replaced simultaneously, and that didn't keep him from leaving the hospital on crutches the next day.

He figures he had no choice but to do both hips. "Both legs were the bad leg," he says.

Eric, a medical doctor, knew he suffered from an unusual condition known as "femoral-acetabular impingement syndrome," which grinds off the cartilage in the hip joint. Aside from producing pain, it eventually leads to loss of hip motion. Eric describes it as, "A gnawing, aching feeling. I struggled to put on shoes." A division-one tennis player in college, he was forced by mounting pain to give up cherished sports in his late 20s—first basketball, then soccer, and finally, tennis.

He tried arthroscopic surgery, but it failed to make his hips feel right. After reviewing his x-rays, Dr. Moschetti told him his hips suffered from advanced arthritis and recommended replacing both of them. Faced with a limited, declining quality of life, Eric decided to proceed with surgery.

At Eric's request, Moschetti operated with spinal anesthesia and a sedative, though general anesthesia was normal for dual hip surgery. Like me, Eric had hoped to be released from the hospital the day of surgery, but wasn't ready. Having lost a lot of blood, he almost passed out when he first sat up.

He rallied quickly, however. That night, he hobbled around the ward on crutches. He didn't like walkers, and found his hips tolerated his weight if both legs shared his weight with crutches. Instead of a three-point crutch footprint, he left a four-point footprint.

He was released the next day, started physical therapy three days later and never looked back. At the end of a week, he hobbled up the Mt. Tom carriage road on crutches for 25 minutes, and was exhausted. Another week later, he dropped the crutches and walked to the top of that little peak. Moschetti heard about it, Eric recalls, and, "I got a stern talking-to—not to be stupid."

The temptation to do more was strong. "Nothing was painful," says Eric. "It seemed like every day I was able to do something more." So he pushed it. He went back to work and danced much of the night after four weeks. After six weeks, he kite-boarded off Cape Cod.

Still, there were times he had to back off. He recalls being overcome by the need to take a nap in the middle of the day. "The thing I wasn't really expecting was how much surgery knocks you out."

Months later, back at work on his three-year-long cardiology fellowship, Eric wonders how long his new hips will last; but isn't worried. "I'd like to get 20 years out of them," he says. But if he has to do the surgery again in ten years, he says, that will be okay. "I'll be back to work after a month."

Three months after surgery, Eric finally played tennis again. He was not as fast as he used to be, but it felt good to be playing. The ski season was next, he said. "I'm looking forward to seeing what I can do in three or four more months."

~

32

TRAVEL TIPS

For most people, modern air travel has gone from a luxury to an ordeal. Seat space has shrunk, security screening has expanded, delays have become chronic. My pre-surgery briefing papers included tips on how to prevent blood clots forming while traveling. Though written for joint replacement patients, they appear useful for travelers in general, especially older ones.

The first, and least practical, advice was to keep your feet elevated. That might work in some first class or business class sections, but is almost impossible back in the economy section, where I fly. As a fallback, my sheet suggested I rest my feet on my carry-on luggage.

The second, and more useful, suggestion was to get up and move about the cabin. I had made that a habit for air travel anyway.

My instructions included the following exercises:

- ankle circles
- foot pumps
- knee lifts

- shoulder rolls
- arm curls.

Also recommended were a series of stretches, which I won't bore you with, but which are also a good idea to keep blood flowing and joints from stiffening.

For me, air travel did produce one disappointment. I thought my new metal hip parts would set off the metal detectors of the federal government's Transportation Safety Administration. They didn't. On my first flight, I proudly announced I had metal in my hip, and was diverted to a pat-down. On my return flight, I decided to see what happened with the metal detector, and I went through without setting off an alarm. From TSA's Web site comments, I gather it is not uncommon for metal hips and knees to pass through without alarms. It may depend on the sensitivity setting on the scanner.

33

STICKER SHOCK—AND RECOVERY

When I was preparing for surgery, I asked DHMC's financial office what it would cost. The bean-counters told me that the out-of-pocket cost for a Medicare patient like me would be about $1,700. That sounded pretty reasonable, especially since I had supplementary insurance that might pay some of that.

But, I added, what about the charges to Medicare? I cared about the bills I ran up for the government program. The answer was, "about $52,000."

I went into shock. How, I asked myself, could they justify that kind of charge?

The answer was much less shocking, but lay tangled in the byzantine billing practices of modern American medicine. As it turned out, the hospital billed a little over $45,000; but after Medicare got finished disallowing about half of it, DHMC collected less than $21,000, mostly from Medicare. My supplement plan chipped in about what the hospital said I would owe. Another $1,200 was billed by my physical therapist; but he got only a little over half that in payments from my insurers.

So my advice to patients is, be prepared to see big numbers. The hospitals know their charges will get down-sized by Medicare. They accept the bill-trimming as part of the game.

I have no complaints. When the financial smoke cleared, I realized that I personally had paid about $30 for my new hip. I had just paid our veterinarian five times that much to treat Hyper Piper, one of our border collies, for a cut on her paw.

HOW LONG WILL IT LAST?

I was 70 at the time of my surgery. Moschetti told me I am likely to wear out before my artificial hip joint does. The plastic liner in my acetabulum cup can wear down, but improvements in polyethylene durability have cut that erosion to an extremely low rate.[42] The stem and cup can get loosened, but that's rare too.

Younger hip replacement patients have more reason to worry they'll outlive their new joints. Scott, who got new hips in his 50s, is expecting to have to redo one or the other eventually. So is Eric, who was 30 when his hips were replaced. Not only do younger hip replacement patients have longer to live, but they also tend to be more active and wear out parts more rapidly.

But their hips might go the distance too. The fact is there isn't very good evidence on how long hip joints last. The few long-term studies are impaired by the fact that most people getting hips replaced are over 65, so the years they use the joints are limited by mortality. Joint products also evolve, which means the new models' survivability has not been tested long. DHMC told me that 80 to 85 percent of implants are still working after 20 years. The longest studies I could find suggested that for one long-used type of hip joint product, more than 80 percent were still working fine after 23 years.[43] If we assume products have improved since that model came out, survivorship should have, too.

PATIENT #11: STEPH

ADVERSE REACTIONS TO MEAL DEBRIS

~

S teph had both hips replaced—*twice.*

Steph is a law professor who used to ride in occasional fox hunts near her home in rural Virginia and took her family kayaking in Alaska. But in her 50s, arthritis in both hips slowed her down.

"I couldn't ride," she says. "I was headed for a wheelchair. I was in agony."

After she got one hip replaced, the pain on that side went away. It was so successful, she decided to get her other hip done before its pain got worse. She hardly used the narcotic that doctors prescribed for her. She was delighted with the results. Within six months she was hiking and riding.

But after a few years, hip problems crept back into her life. She was notified that if the implants had been improperly installed they could cause problems. Her doctor said hers looked good. Yet she didn't feel good. "For two years, I felt terrible... all over... Everything ached." She found a series of stories in the New York Times about problems caused by the same implants she had received. People were getting sick because the implants' metal sockets and metal ball joints shed particles and ions of metal into surrounding tissues and the blood stream.

She went back to her doctor, saying, "I feel like I've aged 100 years." A blood test showed cobalt concentrations so high that Steph called them, "off the charts."

The metal-on-metal joints had been promoted for athletic, younger patients. They enabled doctors to put in a larger ball joint that would resist dislocation better and last longer than smaller joints with plastic liners. But adverse reactions to metal debris sickened and damaged some people.

She got both hip joints replaced again, getting plastic liners and ceramic heads. Metal particles had caused pseudotumors in her hips that were so bad, Steph said, the surgeon didn't want to delay the second hip. Doctors replaced it only two weeks after the first.

She is not alone. Makers of metal-on-metal hip joints have been swamped by lawsuits from patients claiming painful injury. Industry leader Johnson & Johnson agreed to pay $2.5 billion to settle claims from some 8,000 patients and discontinued a leading metal-on-metal hip joint. Several countries issued health warnings about such devices, and their use has declined sharply. Lawsuits continue.

Steph recovered quickly. Within four months after replacement surgery she walked her home town's annual 10-kilometer racecourse. One of the winning runners was so impressed he gave her his prize.

Still, she hasn't recovered fully. She had always relied on strong legs to keep her seat on a horse when it wheeled, bucked or shied. Tumors have weakened her legs. She is more prone to fall off. She still rides, but has given up raucous fox hunts for placid trail rides. She puts a strap around her horse's neck, which she can grab if she's losing her seat.

Though it's been difficult and painful, Steph says she has no regrets about getting hip surgery. "I was in agony before" the surgeries, she recalled. "I'm much better off than if I had done nothing."

~

35

THE BIG TEST

The hike had long been at the top of my bucket list: Torres del Paine National Park, where granite peaks spring skyward from the southern tip of South America. Jagged crags and vertical towers make it distinctive, and incredibly scenic. I called it the Grand Tetons on steroids.

Toni had given me a trip there as a birthday present a few years ago, but my hip pain kept us from booking it. Now my new hip seemed strong and comfortable—but would it be up to that much hiking?

An online adventure-travel fixer booked us into the four-day "W-trek", so-called because it inscribes a W around the southern contours of the mountains with an ascent north into the heart of them in the midst of the tour. We'd stay in communal shelters called refugios. They'd provide beds and meals, so we wouldn't have to carry tents, sleeping bags or food. They were about ten miles apart and were booked months in advance, so we'd have to average more than ten miles per day, with no days off or freedom to change our itinerary. I'd done that kind of hiking on the Appalachian

Trail with more weight in my pack, and I'd done day hikes since the surgery. But I didn't know if the new hip would rebel against multi-day trekking.

We scheduled the trip for February, the austral summer, nine months after my hip got replaced. By then, I figured, most of the disturbed tissues should be fully healed, even in an old fogey like me. Fortunately, the trail stayed below 3,000 feet in elevation. Climbing and descending would be moderate. And I lightened my load by weeding out stuff I might not need.

Toni was another concern. She had overcommitted herself into volunteer activities at home, as usual, and couldn't find time to practice carrying her full pack even one day (which was all I found time for). Yet she and I walked dogs a couple of miles per day, and did a spinning class twice a week for about six weeks. I read a book about this hike by a woman who got ready by hiking with a pack for months. When I told Toni, she shrugged it off. "I'm strong," she said. "I can do it."

In the end, we couldn't be sure how we'd do. We'd have to just do it and find out.

The trek started awkwardly. We were supposed to take a boat up Grey Lake to the foot of a massive glacier, where we were due to go kayaking and settle into our first refugio. But gale-force winds and rain cancelled the first sailing. By the time we got up the lake on the early afternoon boat, we had missed the kayaking.

From there, the weather gods smiled on us. We had four days of great hiking in everything from calm sunshine to clouds and the region's trademark 50 mile-per-hour winds, but never more than a sprinkling of rain. We passed turquoise lakes, rainbows, ghost forests (bleached trunks left by a wildfire) and night stars the size of snowballs. Refugios were cramped but surprisingly comfortable and reverberated with a babel of languages.

We did 12-plus miles the first day, which was a bit of a slog. But the days got easier. Toni had a painful toe and I developed a heel blister. I did take some naproxen, the anti-inflammatory drug, to ward off any pains, but I probably didn't need to. To my delight, my hip never gave me a single twinge.

The highlight came the last morning. We rose at 4:15 and hiked two hours by headlamps up through forest and steep boulders. We reached the park's namesake towers in the faint glow of dawn, praying that no clouds would block the sunrise. Dozens of hikers huddled in the rocks, waiting. Between 6:30 and 7:00: the sun peeked over the horizon and bathed the towers in pink—then red.

Thank you, Dr. Moschetti.

36

APPENDIX ONE

I n the Operating Room
I couldn't resist observing hip replacements in Dr. Moschetti's operating room. The procedure looked more like carpentry than medicine. We're talking about drills, saws and hammers; reamers, planers and screws. The main difference between Moschetti's tools and those in my garage was the hospital's antiseptic preference for polished metal.

You can find videos and animations of surgeries on YouTube and on some hospital and medical devices Web sites. If you're squeamish about the sight of blood, stick with the animations and skip the videos—and my following description. But if you're interested in how doctors replace a hip joint, allow me to walk you through an anterior total hip replacement that I watched over Moschetti's shoulder.

First, consider the physics. The hip is a ball and socket joint. The head of your thigh bone, or femur, is ball-shaped. It turns within a cup-like socket in the pelvis called the acetabulum. Both of these structures are covered in soft cartilage, which provides a cushion over the bone, but also hosts nerves that register pain. Strong muscles hold the two together.

OA occurs when the cartilage wears off the ball-shaped femoral head and the acetabulum. Without that cartilage, bone rubs against bone, causing pain. Often, rough bone spurs increase pain and grinding. The ball's shape is no longer round. Think of a lemon in a spherical hole; it doesn't rotate smoothly.

Here's what the hip replacement surgery looked like to me:

Outside the operating room, Moschetti, his physician assistant and resident don helmets that suspend a light from their foreheads. They wear heavy lead aprons to protect them from radiation from using x-ray. They scrub their arms and hands vigorously with soap, water and a scrub brush. Over their blue "scrub" shirts and pants, nurses clad them in blue gowns and slip head dresses with clear facial shields over their head gear. They're helped into not just one, but two pairs of sterile gloves. That completes their sterile "space suit." They look a little like astronauts exploring the moon.

All this protective equipment is designed to shield them from blood—which will soon spatter on them—and the patient from infection.[44] Only about one in 100 hip replacement patients gets an infection, but it's an ugly problem that everyone wants to avoid. Metal doesn't have blood vessels, so all the antibiotic you can put in the blood stream may not cure an infection on a joint replacement. If drugs can't kill the infection, treatment then relies on removing all the metal from the bone, killing off the infection and starting over. This presents a challenge as the bone actually grows into, or is cemented to, the skin of the metal implants.

Moschetti's patient is sedated after a spinal anesthetic

numbs her legs. She's lying on her back under moveable lights, surrounded by rolling tables of medical tools and a portable x-ray machine called a C-arm. Flat screen monitors near her head show her vital signs. Anesthesiologist Brian Sites, in blue scrubs, watches them. Bags of saline solution and medications drip into clear plastic tubes plugged into her veins.

Her feet are placed in what looks like ski boots and she is transferred supine onto a table that is specially designed for anterior hip surgery. It has movable extensions that allow the surgeons to raise, lower, open, close and turn the legs as required by the surgery. It might have come in handy in medieval times, when drawing and quartering was a popular technique of torture and execution. Today it has more beneficial uses.

To guard the patient against infection, she is rubbed from chest to feet, first with alcohol to kill any bacteria on the skin and then with an iodine and alcohol based paint. The team covers her with sterile blue drapes that are secured with adhesive tape. Gradually the human form disappears under protective coatings. Only two windows are left: one for her head and another for her right hip which is now covered with an iodine-impregnated drape which adheres to the skin. The check-list begins. All members of the team introduce themselves, the patient is identified, the surgical site and procedure are confirmed and several other items are "checked". Piercing the adherent drape, Moschetti injects the area with a numbing local anesthetic. It's time to start cutting.

Moschetti makes the first incision with a scalpel. Once inside the epidermis, the surgeons do most of their cutting with an electric cautery device called a bovie, which simultaneously cuts through tissue and stops bleeding. A large roll of plastic, like a large condom with two open ends, is inserted in the wound. It serves as another layer of infection control around the edges of the incision, protects the skin and helps metal "retractors" separate tissues. A suction tube vacuums blood out of the wound, and the team frequently mops up blood with gauze pads and cauterize tissue to decrease blood loss. I am amazed there isn't more bleeding.

Working smoothly, surgeons inject more numbing medication. They cut through fascia that looks a little like plastic wrap, and yellow globs of fat. Surgeons clamp two blood vessels. Their large, stainless steel retractors move aside red muscles and other tissues until they see the hip "capsule," a sac that encloses the hip joint and contains fluid that lubricates it. Slicing open the capsule, they have arrived.

The surgical approach to the joint happens fast. I hear the saw buzz. The neck of the femur is being cut to remove the arthritic head. The next thing I know the resident has corkscrewed a long-handled tool into the head of the femur. Next he's trying to wrench it out. He's twisting it and pulling on it hard, with both hands, and it's not coming.

"C'mon Mike!" prods Moschetti.

Something gives way. Mike holds aloft what looks a little like a cue ball.

"Look at that," someone comments. "There's no cartilage on that head." Which was the reason the patient needed surgery.

The first step to building a new joint is to make a new socket. Moschetti asks for a two-handed, drill-like reamer with a hemisphere-shaped rasp. He steers it into the hole in the patient's hip, placing it in the acetabulum (the socket in the pelvis). He leans into the reamer as it rotates, carving worn out cartilage from the socket. He goes on to a larger reamer, then another.

"Let's go to a 51," he says, ordering the reamer one size smaller than the cup that he wants to implant. The cup is a partial hemisphere of metal with several holes, through which screws can be driven, and a rough, porous outer surface into which bone is supposed to grow. The actual implant is slightly larger than the last reamer so it will stay in place when surgeons wedge it into the pelvis socket.

Inserting a test cup, Moschetti wheels over the C-arm x-ray machine to check its location and angle. It's not quite right. Removing the cup, he manually scrapes some material from the socket with a long, sharp curette. Finally, using a long-handled tool, he carefully places the metal cup into the socket. Taking a stainless-steel hammer, he whacks it into place.

To secure the cup, Moschetti drills a hole through it into the pelvis and drives a screw into the hole. This is more difficult than it sounds. He's working with an articulated screw driver designed to drive a screw at an angle at the bottom of a narrow opening in a human body. After putting in a second screw, he inserts a plastic liner that locks into the metal shell. The socket is done.

Soon, Moschetti is looking at the open end of the thigh bone (the upper end of the now-headless femur). Like bones we've seen dogs chew, it looks like a misshapen pipe, roughly an oval of white bone with a partly hollow, marrow-lined center. "Lower leg," Moschetti commands. One of the attendants manipulates the table; moving the leg down and turning it out 125 degrees. I grimace, but remind myself that the leg bones are no longer attached to the pelvis

Moschetti starts with a small metal "broach," a file-like wedge that widens from a point to a diameter comparable to the bone's interior and resembles the shape of the actual stem that he'll implant in the femur. He inserts the broach into the top of the femur and hammers it in.

He whacks the first broach hard. Fitting the stem in the femur isn't a delicate process. After it fits snugly, he taps upward on a side wing of the broach to loosen and remove it. He hammers in two or three progressively larger broaches, widening the hole inside the femur. At times, he drops the hammer and takes up a drill with a horizontal planer. With that, he files down the bone from the top of the femur so that the final stem will sit flush with the bone. When he gets a tight fit with the broach of the correct size he mounts a trial stem and blue trial ball on the femur, puts it in the socket and checks it out on a portable x-ray image.

Moschetti uses a computer program before surgery to estimate the size of the implants which best match each individual's skeleton. The goal is to restore the patient's anatomy using an implant which matches the individual's bone in shape and size.

The fluoroscope shows the stem going in at more of an angle than Moschetti likes, so he adjusts. He dislocates the hip, removes the test implants. He planes, hammers, moves to a different stem, and x-rays again.

Finally, he's satisfied. The x-ray shows the stem fitting vertically in the femur, as it should. Moschetti hammers home the stem and locks a shiny metal ball on its top. The team lifts and rotates the leg into position and puts the ball in the socket.

"I decided to go with a bigger stem," he explained later.

It's important to get the size right. If the stem is too small, it can sink down too far in the bone (subside) or get loose. If the stem is loose and the bone doesn't grow to the metal the patient will have pain. One risk of going too big is that he might crack or split the femur.

"How do you know how hard you can drive it in?" I ask. After doing hundreds of operations, Moschetti says he gets a feel for this. If he makes a mistake and cracks a bone, he secures a wire around the bone to hold it together, but his mistakes are rare.

It sounds relatively simple. It's not. Surgeons have to deal with many complexities, among them: avoiding infection, controlling bleeding, using the right sized reamers and broaches to make the cup and stem fit, firmly seating the cup in the right configuration, matching the cup and ball, getting the surgical leg-length as close as possible to that of the other leg. They have to work in a small hole into a living body using cutting tools, reamers, drills, an articulated screw driver, while making sure not to cut into a major artery or nerve, which could be devastating.

The payoff is huge. As they throw away damaged femoral heads, skilled surgeons like Moschetti toss out a life of pain and disability. Their patients start to walk the day of their surgery.

APPENDIX TWO

Your Results May Vary
   I am offering this account in hopes that others can learn something from my experiences and those of my friends and acquaintances. My doctor emphasized that every person is different; I should be cautious about generalizing from my own experience. So in the spirit of full disclosure, here's where I came from.

Some hip replacement patients are already pretty handicapped when they go in for the surgery; I was not. At 70, I was well past middle age, but I was active. As an adult, I had indulged in running, skiing, biking, hiking and anything else that would help me stay in shape. In my 60's, my younger son, Lee, lured me into playing with his men's ice hockey team. I was pretty bad, but this wasn't the NHL. He and my older son, Grant, also got me into sprint triathlons, which were a challenge, because I swam like a brick. But they helped keep me in shape.

I had always been on the skinny side. And I was lucky; I'd never had to deal with diabetes or heart disease, like some close friends. I didn't smoke. I didn't drink much. My worst addiction was to chocolate chip cookies.

My attributes tend to correlate with good hip replacement outcomes, yet I'm convinced my recovery wasn't unusual. In interviewing hip patients, I was impressed by how quickly and close to completely most of them recovered. To be sure, most of the hip patients I interviewed had also been active adults. Their age at surgery ranged from the 30s to the 80s. Their intensity varied from Eric, the tennis player and Neil, the obsessive mountain hiker, to Roseanne and Camilla, who'd long been hobbled by a bad knee and ankle, respectively. The latter two had some of the toughest recoveries in this book, but that was partly due to other injuries and conditions.

This was a diverse pool of patients, and they all had good surgical outcomes. If you're an active adult in relatively good shape, it's likely you can too.

(One note about the patient stories: these accounts came from interviews with patients, not their doctors. I cannot vouch for the medical accuracy of their descriptions of their procedures, symptoms and complications. This is how they described them to me.)

EPILOGUE

FOOTNOTES LISTED BY CHAPTER

T he software I have used to publish this book does not permit me to insert footnotes at the foot of each page. I found medical literature useful in researching the topics in this volume. So, to show some of these sources and help readers who want to do their own research, I have listed below footnotes that give sources for some of the text. The number for each footnote is found in the text as a small, elevated number, like this: [45]. I have listed them below by the chapter in which they appear. Most of these refer to medical papers that can be found by pasting the titles into the National Library of Medicine's Web site, easily found at www.PubMed.gov. A few of these footnotes simply give scientific names for tissues that are described colloquially in the text.

Introduction

1 Cary MP, et al.: Changes in Payment Regulation and Acute Care Use for Total Hip Replacement: Trends in

Length of Stay, Costs, and Discharge, 1997–2012. Rehabil Nurs. 2016 March; 41(2): 67–77. doi:10.1002/rnj.210.

CHAPTER One

2 Simon Dagenais, DC, PhD,1,2 Shawn Garbedian, MD,1 and Eugene K. Wai, MD, MSc1, Systematic Review of the Prevalence of Radiographic Primary Hip Osteoarthritis, Clin Orthop Relat Res. 2009 Mar; 467(3): 623–637.

3 Kurtz S, Ong K, Lau E, Mowat F, Halpern M. Projections of primary and revision hip and knee arthroplasty in the United States from 2005 to 2030. J Bone Joint Surg Am. 2007 Apr, 89(4): 780-5

4 Wolford ML, Palso K and Bercovitz A. Hospitalization for Total Hip Replacement Among Inpatients Aged 45 and Over: United States, 2000-2010. NCHS Data Brief No. 186, February 2015

CHAPTER Two

5 interview, Moschetti W, 7/14/2017

6 Cleveland Clinic, Men's Health Advisor, Vol. 19, Number 8, August 2017

7 Goldstein JP[1, et al.].The Cost and Outcome Effectiveness of Total Hip Replacement: Technique Choice and Volume-Output Effects Matter. Appl Health Econ Health Policy. 2016 Dec;14(6):703-718

8 Jasvinder A. Singh, MBBS, MPH,[1] C. Kent Kwoh, MD,[2] Robert M. Boudreau, PhD,[2] Gwo-Chin Lee, MD,[3] and Said A. Ibrahim, MD, MPH[2,3], Hospital volume and surgical outcomes after elective hip/knee arthroplasty: A risk adjusted analysis of a large regional database. Arthritis Rheum. 2011 Aug; 63(8): 2531–2539.

doi: 10.1002/art.30390

9 Wojciechowski P[1], et al. Minimally invasive approaches in total hip arthroplasty. Ortop Traumatol Rehabil. 2007 Jan-Feb;9(1):1-7.

10 Katz JN, et al. Association Between Hospital and Surgeon Procedure Volume and Outcomes of Total Hip Replacement in the United States Medicare Population. J Bone Joint Surg Am. 2001 Nov;83-A(11):1622-9.

Chapter Four

11 Posterior surgery cuts the piriformis and superior gemeli muscles.

12 Demos HA, et al, Instability in primary total hip arthroplasty with the direct lateral approach. Clin Orthop Relat Res. 2001 Dec;(393):168-80.

13 Direct anterior surgery operates between the rectus femoris and tensor faciae latae muscles.

14 Four-fold lower dislocation claim comes from DePuy Synthes Institute Web site (maker of artificial hip components).

15 Udai S. Sibia, MD, MBA, et al., The Impact of Surgical Technique on Patient Reported Outcome Measures and Early Complications After Total Hip Arthroplasty, The Journal of Arthroplasty 32 (2017) 1171e1175

16 Higgins, BT, et al., 2015, Anterior vs. posterior approach for THA, a systematic review and meta-analysis, The Journal of Arthroplasty 2015, 419-434

17 Meermans G[1], Konan S[2], Das R[2], Volpin A[2], Haddad FS[3] The direct anterior approach in total hip arthroplasty: a systematic review of the literature. Bone Joint J. 2017 Jun;99-B(6):732-740. doi: 10.1302/0301-620X.99B6.38053.

18 The nerve to the outer thigh is the lateral femoral cutaneous nerve.

19 Anterior surgery history from DePuy Synthes Institute (maker of artificial hip components) Web site.

Chapter Seven

20 Basques BA[1], et al., General compared with spinal anesthesia for total hip arthroplasty.

J Bone Joint Surg Am. 2015 Mar 18;97(6):455-61. doi: 10.2106/JBJS.N.00662.

Chapter Eight

21 US Department of HHS, NCHS Data Brief No. 186, February, 2015

22 Molloy IB et al., Effects of the Length of Stay on the Cost of Total Knee and Total Hip Arthroplasty from 2002 to 2013. J Bone Joint Surg Am. 2017 Mar 1;99(5):402-407. doi: 10.2106/JBJS.16.00019.

23 Cleveland Clinic, Men's Health Advisor, Vol. 19, Number 8, August 2017

24 Sibia US et al., Predictors of Hospital Length of Stay in an Enhanced Recovery After Surgery Program for Primary Total Hip Arthroplasty, The Journal of Arthroplasty 31 (2016) 2119e2123

Chapter Eleven

25 Mantilla CB[1], Horlocker TT, Schroeder DR, Berry DJ, Brown DL. Frequency of myocardial infarction, pulmonary embolism, deep venous thrombosis, and death

following primary hip or knee arthroplasty. Anesthesiology. 2002 May;96(5):1140-6.

Chapter Twelve

26 Cleveland Clinic, Men's Health Advisor, Vol. 19, Number 8, August 2017

CHAPTER THIRTEEN

27 Davis MA, et al., Prescription Opioid Use Among Adults with Mental Health Disorders in the United States, J Am Board Fam Med. 2017 Jul-Aug;30(4):407-417. doi: 10.3122/jabfm.2017.04.170112.

28 National Academies of Sciences, Engineering and Medicine: Pain Management and the Opioid Epidemic: Balancing Societal and Individual Benefits and Risks of Prescription Opioid Use, July 13, 2017

29 Chang AK, Bijur PE, Esses D, Barnaby DP, Baer J. Effect of a Single Dose of Oral Opioid and Nonopioid Analgesics on Acute Extremity Pain in the Emergency DepartmentA Randomized Clinical Trial. JAMA. 2017;318(17):1661–1667. doi:10.1001/jama.2017.16190

30 Demetrios N. Kyriacou, MD, PhD[1,2], Opioid vs Nonopioid Acute Pain Management in the Emergency Department, JAMA. 2017;318(17):1655-1656. doi:10.1001/jama.2017.16725

CHAPTER EIGHTEEN

31 Momaya AM, et al., Return to Driving After Hip Arthroscopy, Clin J Sport Med 2017;0:1-5

32 Qurashi S et al., Driving After Microinvasive Total Hip Arthroplasty, J Arthroplasty. 2017 May;32(5):1525-1529.

33 Abbas G, et al., Resumption of car driving after total hip replacement. J Orthop Surg (Hong Kong). 2011Apr;19(1):54-6.

34 Van der Velden CA, et al., When is it safe to resume driving after total hip and total knee arthroplasty? a meta-analysis of literature on post-operative brake reaction times. Bone Joint J. 2017 May;99-B(5):566-576. doi: 10.1302/0301-620X.99B5.BJJ-2016-1064.R1.

Chapter Twenty-two

35 Issa K[1], et al., Sexual Activity After Total Hip Arthroplasty: A Systematic Review of the Outcomes. J Arthroplasty. 2017 Jan;32(1):336-340.

CHAPTER TWENTY-EIGHT

36 Newman JT[1] et al. Return to Elite Level of Play and Performance in Professional Golfers After Arthroscopic Hip Surgery. Orthop J Sports Med. 2016 Apr 18;4(4):2325967116643532. doi: 10.1177/2325967116643532. eCollection 2016 Apr.

CHAPTER THIRTY

37 Murphy L, et al., The impact of osteoarthritis in the United States: a population-health perspective. Am J Nurs. 2012 Mar;112(3 Suppl 1):S13-9. doi: 10.1097/01.NAJ.0000412646.80054.21.

38 Dagenais S, et al. Systematic Review of the Prevalence of Radiographic Primary Hip Osteoarthritis

Clin Orthop Relat Res. 2009 Mar; 467(3): 623–637.

39 op. cit., Cary MP et al.

40 op. cit., Murphy L et al.

41 Ibid, Murphy L et al.

CHAPTER THIRTY-FOUR

42 Devane, Peter A. et al., Highly Cross-Linked Poly-ethylene Reduces Wear and Revision Rates in Total Hip Arthroplasty: A 10-Year Double-Blinded Randomized Controlled Trial. JBJS: October 18, 2017 - Volume 99 - Issue 20 - p 1703–1714; doi: 10.2106/JBJS.16.00878

43 Vidalain, Jean-Pierre, Twenty-year results of the cementless Corail stem. International Orthopaedics (SICOT) (2011) 35:189–194 DOI 10.1007/s00264-010-1117-2

Appendix One

44 Bryan D. Springer, et al., Infection burden in total hip and knee arthroplasties: an international registry-based perspective. Arthroplasty Today 3 (2017) 137e140

AFTERWORD

Being an orthopaedic surgeon is an incredible privilege. Every day I wake up and think about how fortunate I am to have a job where I can help people in such an impactful and enjoyable way. In essence, my job entails taking people's physical pain away. For me that comes in the form of hip and knee arthritis. Simply, with surgery I remove the arthritic old parts and replace them with new parts. Those new parts are typically made of metal and plastic. This reliably can diminish pain and restore function for someone debilitated by arthritis. Seeing the improvement patients experience after surgery is really the most satisfying part of my job. Joint replacement is a life-changing procedure and it is an honor to have patients entrust me with their bodies.

Despite performing hundreds of joint-replacement operations a year, I always place my focus on each individual patient. In medicine, we can place people into groups based on health characteristics and comorbidities but truly, everyone is different. This might be the first surgery ever for someone, which may be overwhelming, or it could just be another procedure for someone with a more complicated history. Everyone has their own preconceived notion of what surgery will be like and what to expect, based on past personal experiences and encounters they have had with others. This, in part, is why we ask all our patients to attend our "joints class" prior to undergoing surgery.

The class is an opportunity for our nurses and physical therapist to provide information to patients on what to expect throughout their joint replacement journey. I have begun to include myself as part of the class, giving a 30-minute presentation on the specifics of hip and knee replacement, as well as the risks and benefits of surgery. Certainly, I thought this was more than enough information to get any patient through their surgery. That was until I met Rob Taylor.

Rob attended the joints class with his notebook in hand jotting down all the information he thought relevant. I then met with him in clinic after the class on a one-on-one basis and asked if he had any questions. The way the system is intended to work, and does most of the time, is that we have answered all the questions a patient could think of. Thus, the usual response to my questions is, "no, you've covered everything thoroughly in the class." Rob was different. He asked if I could point him to any resources written from the patient's perspective and not provided by medical personnel. I unfortunately could not. He then told me he was a writer and that he might put something together. I could see the wheels turning in his head and knew he was serious.

I can describe Rob as the ideal patient. Active and healthy with minimal medical issues, didn't smoke, thin with good anatomy, taking minimal pain meds for severe arthritis, motivated and engaged. He's the kind of patient you sense is just going to do well. There is good evidence that patients who smoke, have diabetes, who are taking pre-operative narcotic pain medication, and who have mental illness tend to have worse outcomes after elective joint replacement, and surgery in general, for that matter. Taking care of Rob thus was a piece of cake. One of my biggest concerns for patients like Rob though is slowing them down. When arthritis pain gets better after surgery it is not uncommon for a patient to overdo it and call with increasing pain. I tell all patients it can take a year to eighteen months to fully recover after a joint replacement. This is a bone surgery and not a soft-tissue surgery. The soft tissues around the joint; muscles, tendons and ligaments, need time to recovery after surgery and this takes time. With a stiff arthritic joint, the muscles lose their flexibility and get weak. It takes time after surgery for these to recover. Commonly I get calls after surgery that "my hip was good for the first few weeks and now it's hurting more." When probed further on their activity patients will confess to stacking two cords of wood, snow-blowing their driveway, walking 18 holes of golf, etc. Despite the arthritis pain going away the muscles, tendons and ligaments need more time to recover and are just not ready for that level of activity very quickly. I will tell patients that what they need, in addition to their prescriptions for pain medicine and physical therapy, is a prescription for patience. Ice and patience are two of the best things anyone can have after joint replacement surgery.

After surgery, I typically make rounds on the orthopaedic ward to see all my patients. The staffers with whom I make rounds kid me about repeating "my spiel." It's true I say the same thing over and over. I guess that's what happens when you're doing the same thing hundreds of times a year. I remind patients it's a marathon and not a sprint. I tell everyone they're likely to be more sore the second day after surgery than the first. The reason for this is the local anesthetic I use in the surgical wound wears off. The first day sometimes is like the honeymoon day, where patients feel great and can't believe how easy surgery was. Then they get home and get sorer. This is normal. Then, over the ensuing days to weeks they're more active and again may feel even more pain, which again is normal. Elevation, ice, Tylenol and anti-inflammatory medication like naproxen or ibuprofen are crucial to keeping this under control (make sure you check with your own doctor to confirm these medications are safe for you). I did not include narcotic medications here; certainly, there is some role for such pain relievers, but many people can get through a hip replacement without these, which can also have many side effects (constipation, altered mental status, drowsiness, addiction, etc.). Rob was one of those patients.

About the only thing Rob complained about after surgery was that he was given too much pain medication. He was given a medication called Tramadol for pain and I think only used one pill. He was upset that we gave him "so much." Pain medication is a tricky thing. There is no question the opioid epidemic is a real problem wreaking havoc across the country and specifically in New Hampshire, where I practice. We have tried to be very thoughtful about how we prescribe opioids and have recently reviewed the prescribing patterns of our department related to several orthopaedic surgeries, including joint replacement. We found there was a number of pills that could be prescribed, less than what had traditionally been given, which could meet the majority of patients' post-surgical pain needs. Obviously, everyone is different though, and a patient like Rob was at one end of the spectrum while others are at the other end. We are trying to thoughtfully address patient's pain needs and avoid over prescribing narcotic pain meds, which is a challenging problem.

I drew a graph like this for Rob and explained that we are trying to find the spot where we can appropriately treat the majority of patients.

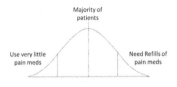

Pain meds needed by a range of patients

Rob was at the far-left end of the graph.

Needless to say, he did well after his hip replacement. His patient reported outcome scores (a score calculated from how he answered questions about his hip and overall health both before and after surgery) improved significantly. He was kayaking with the orcas by summer.

I actually ran into him at the driving range about 6 weeks after surgery, which gave my kids an insight into my work. I took my 6-year-old and 4-year old-sons to the range to hit balls. Initially I was apprehensive when I saw an older man hitting balls by himself. I worry some of the serious golfers don't love little kids, and their dads possibly, hacking it up at the range. As I got closer I realized it was Rob, who greeted me warmly and took an interest in my kids, who were swinging with more enthusiasm than results.

It was great to see a guy who limped into my clinic several weeks earlier out crushing golf balls (keep in mind I was comparing him to my 4- and 6-year-olds). They were curious about him, too and asked how I knew "that guy."

"I gave him a new hip a few weeks ago."

My kids sometimes come in and make rounds with me on the weekends but this was a rare chance to show them the results of my work outside the hospital. They ask me every night at dinner what I did at work. They usually ask, "Was it a helmet day?" (They know I wear a helmet with a headlight in the operating room and think that's the coolest.) I try to explain to them how I help people who have worn-out hips and knees and who can no longer do the things they love to do, like golf, and I give them new parts. This is a high-level concept for a small child to understand. When I visited my son's first grade class to teach them about bones, a child asked me: who needs to get their joints replaced? I simply responded that sometimes when people get older their joints wear out and they need new ones. Another child stated "you should talk to my dad, he's real old and probably needs his joints replaced." In any event Rob made a good advertisement for total hip replacement that even my kids could see. Seventy years of age when he got a new hip, he was still slender and sinewy. That certainly helps the surgery go smoothly. He asked for minimal sedation and discarded most of the narcotic pills we gave him for pain. He made a rapid recovery from surgery, and now he was walking, kayaking, biking and playing golf.

Much like the bell-shaped graph I showed Rob when talking about pain medications I think you could make a similar graph when talking about recovery after hip replacement.

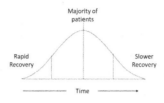

Recovery time varies

Not everyone recovers at the same pace, which is why again I tell patients the full recovery can take a year to eighteen months. That's the point when you will likely stop seeing any improvement in your pain and function. That being said, the vast majority of patients experience the greatest improvement in their pain and function over the first few weeks and months.

The following graph outlines the rapid improvement seen initially followed by slower improvement over time. Keep in mind these are graphs I created to visually display recovery after hip replacement and are meant to be a general guide. I intentionally left a gap at the beginning of the recovery phase as initially after surgery it is common to have good days and bad days before the good days seem to dominate.

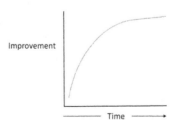

Unfortunately, not everyone who undergoes a joint replacement is always happy with their results and complications can occur. Some people still have some pain after surgery, which may or may not be linked to a definable anatomic cause and in some cases can't be treated. Specifically, hip replacement patients can get an infection, limp, have a discrepancy in their leg lengths (your surgeon can make your leg longer or shorter during the procedure), the prosthetic hip could dislocate (pop out of the joint), the bone could fracture during or after surgery, and there could be injury to major nerves and/or blood vessels. This is not an exhaustive list of complications after surgery and certainly others can occur. Each of them is unlikely, though, and you should ask your surgeon what his or her complication rates are—especially in regards to things like infection, which they and their institution should know. In some cases, these complications can lead to further surgery which could lead to a revision or re-do hip replacement. Revision hip replacement is usually more complicated than the initial surgery and requires a surgeon comfortable taking on these more complex issues. An infection for instance, can be a very big problem and sometimes requires taking the hip replacement out (which is either cemented to the bone or grown to the skeleton and not easy to remove). A good portion of my practice involves revision surgery and it's all too common I hear patients say "I didn't know a problem could occur." This in part is the reason I've focused so much on educating patients through our joints class and where this book can provide beneficial insight.

For most patients though, total hip replacement surgery is a life-changing operation. There are many ways to perform a hip replacement and my bias is towards the anterior approach (replacing the hip through the front of the thigh). There is potentially some short-term benefit to this approach, as it likely does the least amount of damage to muscles. Patients may have less pain in the immediate postoperative period giving them a leg up on the recovery process. But to be honest, any number of approaches to the surgery can be effective in the long run, given a skilled surgeon, an experienced clinic and a little time for the tissues to heal. I tell patients with severe, limiting arthritis that what they need is a well done hip replacement and not an approach. There are pros and cons to all approaches to hip replacement and a well-done surgery by an experienced surgeon will most likely result in a happy patient.

What makes this book unique is that it is written by the patient for the patient. I have enjoyed working with Rob and providing some of my insight but for the most part what you read is Rob's personal account of his hip replacement journey. He's included other stories and perspectives as well, and all of these will prove useful for people who are considering or preparing for a total hip replacement. I have helped him by editing much of the text, allowing him to watch two hip surgeries, providing information during several interview sessions and connecting him with patients who were willing to share their personal hip surgery and recovery experiences. I hope the information provided in this book will act as a helpful resource to those considering total hip replacement.

Wayne E. Moschetti, MD, MS

CPSIA information can be obtained
at www.ICGtesting.com
Printed in the USA
FSHW012015280219
56023FS